Editors **Minoru Ai** ∕ **Yuh-Yuan Shiau**

New Magnetic Applications in Clinical Dentistry

New Magnetic Applications in Clinical Dentistry

Editors

Minoru Ai

Professor Emeritus,
Tokyo Medical and Dental University

Yuh-Yuan Shiau

Professor
Department of Fixed Prosthodontics and Occlusion,
School of Dentistry, National Taiwan University

quintessence
books

Quintessence Publishing Co., Ltd.

Tokyo, Berlin, Chicago, London, Paris, Barcelona, Istanbul, Milano, São Paulo, New Delhi, Moscow, Prague, Warsaw, and Istanbul

Printing and Binding: Sun Art Printing Co., Ltd. Osaka
Printing in Japan
ISBN 4-87417-828-6   C 3047

CONTRIBUTORS

Minoru Ai, DDS, PhD

Professor Emeritus
Tokyo Medical and Dental University
Tokyo, Japan

Yoshinobu Honkura, Dr. Eng

Director
Aichi Steel Corporation
Aichi, Japan

Toshio Hosoi, DDS, PhD

Professor
1st Department of Prosthetic Dentistry,
Tsurumi University, School of Dentistry
Kanagawa, Japan

Tetsuo Ichikawa, DDS, PhD

Professor
Department of Removable Prosthodontics and Oral
Implantology,
The University of Tokushima School of Dentistry
Tokushima, Japan

Yoshimasa Igarashi, DDS, PhD

Professor
Department of Removable Prosthodontics,
School of Dentistry, Matsumoto Dental University
Nagano, Japan

Hiroshi Inoue, DDS, PhD

Professor
Department of Removable Prosthodontics and Occlusion,
Osaka Dental University
Osaka, Japan

Naeko Kawamoto, DDS, PhD

Department of Removable Prosthodontics and Oral
Implantology,
The University of Tokushima School of Dentistry
Tokushima, Japan

Motonobu Miyao, DDS, PhD

Assistant Professor
Department of Oral Functional Science and
Rehabilitation, Division of Prosthodontics,
Asahi University School of Dentistry
Gifu, Japan

Hiroshi Mizutani, DDS, PhD

Assistant Professor
Removable Prosthodontics,
Department of Masticatory Function Rehabilitation,
Division of Oral Health Sciences,
Graduate School, Tokyo Medical and Dental University
Tokyo, Japan

Kazuo Nakamura, DDS, PhD

Sanno Medical Plaza

Organized Center of Clinical Medicine,
International University of Health and Welfare
Tokyo, Japan

Harold W. Preiskel, MDS, MSc, FDS, RCS

Professor Harold Preiskel and Mr. Tim O'Brien
London, England

Vygandas Rutkunas, DDS

Removable Prosthodontics,
Department of Masticatory Function Rehabilitation,
Division of Oral Health Sciences,
Graduate School, Tokyo Medical and Dental University
Tokyo, Japan

Shinsuke Sadamori, DDS, PhD

Assistant Professor
Department of Prosthetic Dentistry,
Division of Cervico-Gnathostomatology,
Graduate School of Biomedical Sciences,
Hiroshima University
Hiroshima, Japan

Yuh-Yuan Shiau, DDS, MS, PhD

Professor
Department of Fixed Prosthodontics and Occlusion,
School of Dentistry, National Taiwan University
Taipei, Taiwan

Seiichiro Someya, DDS

Someya Dental
Tokyo, Japan

Jyoji Tanaka, DDS

Tanaka Dental Clinic
Chiba, Japan

Fujio Tsuchida, DDS

1st Department of Prosthetic Dentistry,
Tsurumi University, School of Dentistry
Kanagawa, Japan

FOREWORD

This book is a new edition of the well-known book, "Construction of Removable Partial Dentures by using Magnetic Attachments" (originally published in Japanese, Quintessence Publishing Co., 1994), which was written by Prof. Minoru Ai of Tokyo Medical and Dental University and his colleagues based on the results of their long years of research and clinical cases using magnetic attachments.

It has long been thought that the forces of attraction or repulsion of magnets could be applied to the fixation of dentures and in actual fact, a number of trials were unsuccessfully made in the 1950s. After persistent efforts were made to study new magnetic materials, rare earth magnets with strong power and small size were developed in the 1970s. Their introduction encouraged the development of retentive appliances for dentures which incorporated these new magnets.

In 1980, Prof. Ai and his research group devised a small magnetic appliance (magnetic attachment) with strong retentive force and high corrosion resistance in the mouth. This device was well accepted in clinical cases. Since then, the magnetic attachment has been improved for practical use due to improvements in its shape and the properties of the built-in magnet, and various types of magnetic attachments are now available for a wide range of applications.

The magnetic attachment is a type of stud attachment used with great success as a retainer for overdentures or removable partial dentures. In 1996, I introduced the magnetic attachment at a meeting of the Asian Chapter of International College of Prosthodontists and it attracted considerable attention from the participants. The International Research Project of Magnetic Dentistry (IRPMD) was established immediately afterwards, and an annual symposium has been held in various countries in Asia, where the latest developments and technical information on magnetic dentistry are actively exchanged. The number of IRPMD members is presently increasing worldwide.

Given this situation, it is most opportune that the basis and clinical cases of the magnetic attachment are explained intensively in this book. It should certainly be helpful for a deeper understanding of this appliance.

The publication of this book is greatly owing to Prof. Ai, who has played a pivotal role in the outstanding achievements of the magnetic attachment, and is also supported by the cooperation of other key IRPMD members. Of particular note are Prof. Yuh-Yuan Shiau of Taiwan University, a great prosthodontist who is fully active in the research and clinical trials of the magnetic attachment, and Prof. Harold Preiskel of London University, a world-famous expert in the research and clinical trials of this attachment. I am quite pleased with the noteworthy contributions of these eminent scholars.

Through this book, readers are expected to gain a better understanding of the magnetic attachment and to provide their patients the benefit of improved clinical technique.

In addition, I would like to mention the IRPMD. The members of this project are researchers of dental universities and dental clinicians in various countries around the world, throughout Asia (Japan, Korea, Taiwan, Hong Kong, China, Thailand, Singapore, Indonesia, Malaysia, India), Europe (U.K., Italy, Germany), and North American (U.S.A., Canada). This book has been supported with the cooperation of the IRPMD members.

Finally, I would like to express my sincere thanks to Dr. Yoshinobu Honkura, Director of Aichi Steel Corporation and all his staff in the Electro-Magnetic Products Division, who continue to offer great support to the IRPMD and generous cooperation in developing the magnetic attachment.

Kenji Hiranuma

President, International Research Project of Magnetic Dentistry

Professor Emeritus, Aichi Gakuin University

and Xian Fourth Military Medical University

PREFACE

The magnetic attachment is a retentive appliance of removable partial dentures. This book presented the philosophy and concepts of the magnetic attachment and its application, and is intended to serve as a reference book for daily dental practice.

For removable partial dentures, retentive appliances are essential. Various types of appliances such as clasps, telescope crowns and attachments have been used. They are requested to work effectively to control the movement of dentures, though the mechanism and function of the retention are different among each other. However, while these appliances work effectively, the abutment teeth are suffering from great stress and sometimes break down due to overstress. In other word, retentive appliances have a positive effect to retain the denture effectively and a negative effect to bring stress on the abutment teeth. How to reduce the negative effect is the most important consideration for designing partial dentures.

The retentive function of the magnetic attachement is based on the attractive force of the magnet built-in. This magnetic function enables the magnetic attachement to have some unique properties, one of which is the control of unfavorable lateral force to the abutment teeth. This leads to the reduction of the negative effect and provides a great advantage which can not be achieved in other retentive appliances. Although the magnetic attachment has to be used only on the devitalized root, however, this can be seen from a different viewpoint as a superior nature, because residual roots can be positively used as abutments of retentive appliance and the periodential tissure can be preserved as well.

The prototype of the magnetic attachment was completed in 1991 and it has been continuously improved and modified thereafter, based on the development of new magnetic materials and the advancement of new technology. Different types of magnetic retentive appliances for removable dentures have been introduced and applied. We belive many more and better magnetic products will be proposed continuously in the future.

In this situation, it is thought significant to compile the basis and clinical applications of the current magnetic attachment intensively into a book.

This book consisted of three parts. In the first part, significance of clinical application of magnet and fundamentals of magnet and magnetic attachment application were discussed. In the second part, technology of magnetic attachment application was introduced. In the third part 27 clinical cases were presented and discussed. Some of them are long-term outcome reports which should encourage the use of the magnetic attachment for clinicians.

The magnetic attachment has been used clinically for more than 10 years, and its advantages and disadvantages are mostly clarified. It is now recognized in general that magnetic attachment is a useful retentive appliance for removable partial prosthesis. Taking clasps and telescope crowns or mechanical attachments as the first and second generation of denture retentive appliances respectively, the magnetic attachement can be regarded as the third generation.

Grateful acknowledgment is expressed to those who devoted great efforts for the development and application of the magnetic attachment. To Mr. Y. Honkura, Phd, Director of Aichi Steel Co. and his staff in the Electromagnetics Division for their ingenious research and development of magnetic attachment. Also, we thank the members of International Research Project of Magnetic Dentistry (IRPMD) for their support and encouragement. Finally, we would like to thank the late Mr. T. Yoshida, editorial director of Quintessence Publishing Co. for his enthusiasm and efforts for publishing this book.

Minoru Ai／Yuh-Yuan Shiau

CONTENTS

Contributors ·· 5
Foreword ··· 7
Preface ··· 9
Contents ··· 11

Chapter 1
Introduction ··· 15
Minoru Ai

Part 1   Fundamentals of Magnet and Magnetic Attachment

Chapter 2
Magnetic Applications in Clinical Dentistry ································ 22
Harold W.Preiskel

Chapter 3
The Technology of the Dental Magnetic Attachment ················· 28
Yoshinobu Honkura

Chapter 4
Biological Effects of Magnetic Attachment on the Human Body and Tissues
·· 44
Tetsuo Ichikawa／Naeko Kawamoto

Chapter 5
Influences of Magnetic Attachment on Medical Appliances ·············· 48
Toshio Hosoi／Fujio Tsuchida

Chapter 6
The New Genaration of Dental Attachment ·························· 51
Yoshinobu Honkura

Part 2　Clinical Application of Magnetic Attachment

Chapter 7
A Concept of Designing Dentures and Role of the Magnetic Attachment
·· 58
Minoru Ai

Chapter 8
Preparations of Abutments for Magnetically Retained Overdentures ······ 70
Hiroshi Mizutani／Vygandas Rutkunas

Chapter 9
Cast base (Coping) system ·· 75
Hiroshi Mizutani／Vygandas Rutkunas

Chapter 10
The Root Keeper System and its Clinical Application ······················ 85
Yuh-Yuan Shiau

Chapter 11
Clinical Analysis on the Reliability of the Magnetic Attachment
over an 8 year period ·· 93
Hiroshi Inoue

Chapter 12
Maintenance of Magnetically Retained Overdentures and Troubleshooting
·· 97
Hiroshi Mizutani／Vygandas Rutkunas

Part 3   Clinical Cases

Case   1 : Replacement of adamaged root surface attachment—1 ·················· 109
Seiichiro Someya

Case   2 : Replacement of adamaged root surface attachment—2 ·················· 111
Hiroshi Mizutani／Vygandas Rutkunas

Case   3 : Replacement of adamaged telescope crown—1 ······················· 114
Motonobu Miyao

Case   4 : Replacement of adamaged telescope crown—2 ······················ 116
Seiichiro Someya

Case   5 : Replacement of adamaged telescope crown—3 ······················ 118
Yoshimasa Igarashi

Case   6 : Replacement of adamaged crown ································ 120
Hiroshi Mizutani／Vygandas Rutkunas

Case   7 : Improvement of poor retention of upper denture ·················· 123
Shinsuke Sadamori

Case   8 : Improvement of poor retention of lower denture—1 ················ 125
Hiroshi Mizutani／Vygandas Rutkunas

Case   9 : Improvement of poor retention of lower denture—2 ················ 127
Seiichiro Someya

Case 10 : Application after extrusion of abutment root ····················· 129
Kazuo Nakamura

Case 11 : Application for short length root—1 ························· 132
Kazuo Nakamura

Case 12 : Application for short length root—2 ························· 134
Kazuo Nakamura

Case 13 : Application for abutment with reduced periodontal support ············ 137
Hiroshi Mizutani／Vygandas Rutkunas

Case 14 : Application for a fractured tooth ·························· 140
Hiroshi Mizutani／Vygandas Rutkunas

Case 15 : Application together with root surface attachment ·················· 143
Hiroshi Mizutani／Vygandas Rutkunas

Case 16 : Application together with telescope crown ·· 146
      Yoshimasa Igarashi

Case 17 : Improvement of crown-root ratio of abutment—1 ······························· 149
      Hiroshi Inoue

Case 18 : Improvement of crown-root ratio of abutments—2 ····························· 153
      Kazuo Nakamura

Case 19 : Improvement of crown-root ratio of abutments—3 ····························· 156
      Hiroshi Mizutani／Vygandas Rutkunas

Case 20 : Reinforcement of stability of upper denture—1 ································· 158
      Hiroshi Mizutani／Vygandas Rutkunas

Case 21 : Reinforcement of stability of upper denture—2 ································· 160
      Hiroshi Mizutani／Vygandas Rutkunas

Case 22 : Improvement of poor appearance of lower denture—1 ····················· 162
      Hiroshi Mizutani／Vygandas Rutkunas

Case 23 : Improvement of poor appearance of lower denture—2 ····················· 164
      Kazuo Nakamura

Case 24 : Improvement of instability and poor appearance of upper denture ······ 166
      Hiroshi Mizutani／Vygandas Rutkunas

Case 25 : Application of the root keeper system ·· 169
      Hiroshi Mizutani／Vygandas Rutkunas

Case 26 : Application for implant supproted lower denture—1 ························· 171
      Jyoji Tanaka

Case 27 : Application for implant supproted lower denture—2 ························· 174
      Jyoji Tanaka

Materials : Dental magnet attachment which are sold in Europe and USA ··················· 178

Index ··· 180

Chapter 1

Introduction

Minoru Ai

The magnetic attachment is a retentive appliance of removable prostheses (*Fig 1*). Numbers of magnetic retentive appliances have been developed, but almost all of them were hardly used because of their low retentive force, corrosion as well as too big size[1, 2]. These problems are completely solved with the magnetic attachment developed in Japan in 1990 and it is making sure of its position as a retainer of dentures[3].

Here, the author would like to mention its significance in the clinical dentistry and the history of its development, and terminology used in this book.

Significance of Magnetic Attachment Applications

The reason why magnetic attachments have spread so rapidly is thought to be in its technical simplicity after all. But, there must have been some advantages in using it or reasonable necessity for it.

Acceptability of Clinical Dentistry for Magnetic Attachments

The magnetic attachment is surely easy to use as a root surface attachment. There are not a few cases where the abutments are destroyed and the retainers can not be used any more. In such cases, the abutments are restored as adjusting to the retainers, or both of abutments and retainers are newly made. Sometimes, the denture itself is remade. But, advent of magnetic attachments make it possible that destroyed parts are repaired easily or instantly by replacement of magnetic

attachments. This is favorable for dentists as well as patients. An advantage is that magnetic attachments can be applied regardless of the path of insertion of dentures. Because of this characteristic, it is possible to use magnetic attachments alone or together with any type of retainers (*Fig 2a, b*). This wide range of its application will be one of the point of its eases to use.

Another point is that residual roots are positively indicated for retention of dentures by using magnetic attachments. Until now, the aim of maintenance of residual roots was mostly for prevention of absorption of the alveolar bone which supports denture bases. By application of magnetic attachments, residual roots came to play a part for retentive effects as well as support of dentures[4].

In addition, magnetic attachments may be used to make dentures useful for the aged and handicapped patients[4, 5]. Dentures with clasps are used in most cases. But, it is sometimes difficult to manage the dentures for disabled hands of those patients. Although the condition is limited such that abutment teeth are required to cut off their crowns, if magnetic attachments are applied for the retainers, the dentures can be easily put in or taken off. This must be very welcomed for helpers as well as patients.

Thus, magnetic attachments have fitted successfully to these deficient parts in conventional clinical dentistry and this will be a real reason why they have come into wide use so rapidly.

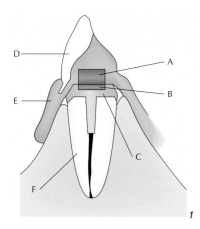

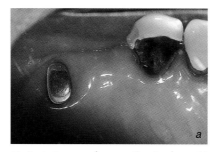

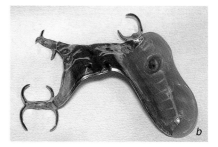

Fig 2a, b A case of magnetic attachment together with clasps (3 years after treatment). a, The keeper in the mouth. b, The denture with magnetic attachment and clasps.

Fig 1 Scheme of magnetic attachment application.
A, Magnetic assembly. B, Keeper. C, Root cap. D, Artificial tooth. E, Denture base. F, Tooth root.

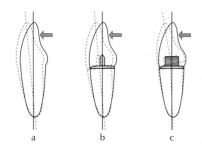

Fig 3 Comparison of the effect of lateral force on the natural tooth root (a), stud attachment and magnetic attachment applied roots (b,c).

Effects of Magnetic Attachments on the Periodontal Tissues

A magnet has such a specific property that its attractive force acts very little in the direction parallel to its attractive surface. This is also a unique property of magnetic attachments having the magnet built-in, which can not be seen in conventional mechanical attachments. With conventional root surface attachments, the lateral force transmitted to the tooth root is little as compared with coronal retainers, and this is favorable to the periodontal tissues. Actually, good results are obtained with root surface attachments. In the case of magnetic attachments, on the other hand, the lateral force which is transmitted to the root through the denture is reduced remarkably according to slide or dislocation of the magnetic attachment on the root surface (Fig 3), and the clinical result is much better than that of mechanical attachments.

This suggests that magnetic attachments can

be used for somewhat mobile teeth as well. In fact, there are some cases to support this[4, 5].

Significance of Preservation of Residual Roots

As mentioned above, residual roots are often preserved in order to use them as the support for sinking of denture bases. But, it involves a great significance in respect of preservation of periodontal ligaments.

In the periodontal ligament, a number of sensory receptors for tactile or pressure sense are included. A pressure brought to the tooth is received by these receptors. The signals from the receptors bring about reflex in the trigeminal nervous system and work for control of jaw movements and occlusal force. Touch to the occlusal surface is perceived through the sensors in the periodontal ligament as occlusal sense and this is related to the taste of foods as a supporter of the sense of taste. In short, sensory receptors in the periodontal ligament has an important role in making jaw function smoothly and improvement of the sense of taste.

Consequently, it should be appreciated that even a residual root which looks valueless at a glance has the periodontal ligaments which play very important role in the control of jaw functions. The tooth root should be preserved in good condition and used effectively. Magnetic attachment application is suitable technique for making good use of such the residual roots.

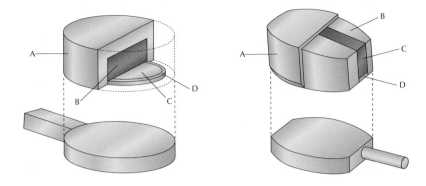

Fig 4a, b Structure of magnetic attachments and the keepers.
a, Cup-yoke type. A, Cup yoke. B, Magnet. C, Disc yoke. D, Ring.
b, Sandwich-yoke type. A, Case. B, Yoke. C, Magnet. D, Spacer.

a | b

Development and Application of Magnetic Attachments

Development of magnetic attachments in Japan was started since about 1980, with introduction of samarium-cobalt magnets. Samarium-cobalt magnet was developed in 1960's and its high magnetism attracted a great attention. Its small size with strong attractive force brought about possibilities of the application of the magnet for clinical dentistry[6].

A small group consisted of researchers of various specialties was organized and real study for the application of the magnet in dental field was started. Focus was placed on bringing the magnet to completion as a root surface attachment. For about 10 years, magnets and magnetic alloys were investigated from various viewpoints of magnetic engineering, biomateriology, physics and biochemistry, as well as clinical applications of magnets.

Influence of Magnetism to Human Body

Influence of magnetism to human body was the most important issue to be cleared. Tissue response and cell growing in the magnetic field were measured. Metal ion solubility, cell toxicity and allergic response on the skin were also tested with magnets and magnetic alloys. The result of every test came up to the national standard. In addition, magnetic flux leakage around magnetic assemblies of completed magnetic attachments was measured. The intensity of the leaked magnetic field was found to be extremely weak com-pared with magnetic appliances used in daily life. This was owing to the closed circuit assemblies.

Reinforcement of Attractive Force

Reinforcement of attractive force of the magnet was also essential problem. Attractive force less than 200gf which was measured with the magnet in the early days was thought to be too small for the retainer of dentures, though suitable retentive force of the retainer was not clarified yet. Only in the conical telescope system, it was determined as 500–600gf.

Advancement of magnets was remarkable and the power was rapidly raised in a short period of time. As for design of magnetic assemblies, it was found that the closed circuit of magnetism, in which magnetic flux was controlled with magnetic alloys (yoke), could make stronger attractive force than the open circuit and the attractive force was influenced with property of yokes and design of assemblage of magnets and yokes.

In 1981, Dr. Gillings[7, 8] reported a new magnetic denture retainer. This was composed of two magnets and a magnetic stainless steel plate as a yoke, which developed a closed circuit of magnetism.

Finally, two types of magnetic assemblies, "cup-yoke type" and "sandwich-yoke type" with the retentive force of 400–450gf were finished[9, 10] (*Fig 4a, b*). The cup-yoke type is such that a cylindrical magnet is set in the cup of magnetic stainless alloy which serves for the yoke, while in the sandwich-yoke type, a cubical magnet is sand-

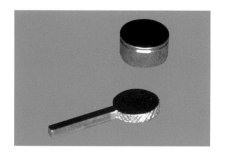 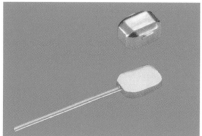

Fig 5a, b Two types of magnetic attachments and the keepers.
a, Cup-yoke type. b, Sandwich-yoke type.

a | b

wiched in between two magnetic stainless alloys as the yoke.

Countermeasure for Corrosion

Rare-earth magnets are easily corroded with saliva in the mouth and lose attractive force. Then, the magnets were to be completely enclosed in anticorrosive stainless steel. A number of stainless steels with different constituents were examined with anticorrosion. Attractive surfaces and yokes of the magnetic assembly were needed to be stainless steels with strong magnetism. But such alloys tended to corrode because of their high content of iron. Strong magnetism and anticorrosion are mostly in reverse relationship, and it was very difficult to find such alloys as satisfying both qualities. Finally, as the power of magnets was expected to rise much more soon, priority was given to the higher anticorrosive property. The magnet was covered with such stainless steel and seams were laser welded.

Completion of Magnetic Attachment

These researches were conducted by the research group in cooperation with two big industrial corporations in Japan, Aichi Steel and Hitachi Metal, which had not related to medical or dental field by the time.

The research group aimed at making such a magnetic appliance that was taken as a genuine retentive appliance, which was safe for human body, effective and widely used in prostheses. The both types of magnetic attachments were tested clinically for several years and various problems concerning appliance itself and its clin-

ical use were properly treated. Effects of the magnetic assembly to medical equipment such as cardiac pacemakers and MRI were also examined.

As the result, magnetic attachments were completed as the root surface attachment, which satisfied all the requirements on retentive force, anticorrosion and clinical use. They were authorized as a medical instrument by Ministry of Health and Welfare of Japan in 1990, and appeared on the market as the name of "Magnetic Attachment" (Fig 5a, b). Their retentive force was 400–600gf acceptable as denture retainers. The research group mostly achieved its aim at the moment, and it was reorganized to the Japanese Society of Magnetic Application in Dentistry (JSMAD) in 1991. Improvement and new development of magnetic attachments were still continued in both corporations and their co-researchers.

New Development of Magnetic Attachment System

The magnet used in the magnetic attachment was changed from samarium-cobalt to neodymium-iron magnet with much stronger attractive force in 1995–96, and the magnetic assembly became smaller and smaller for easy use in clinic. Now, even magnetic attachments with retentive force of 800gf can be obtained. Various types such as stress-breaking or for implant are developed and appeared on the market.

As for the keeper, various trials have been made. But finally, the method to cast a root cap with a ready made stainless steel keeper brought good result in retentive force and avoidance of caries, and it came to a standard.

Recently, new method of the root-keeper system was developed, in which the keeper was fixed directly to the root surface by using adhesive resin and composite resin. It is widely accepted useful for the prosthetic treatment of elderly or handicapped patients without troubles of caries.

Magnetic Attachments at Present and in Future

Now, magnetic attachments have come to be acknowledged as a standard prosthetic retentive appliance. They are used mostly as the retainer of removable partial dentures and overdentures but sometimes in removable bridges or maxillofacial prostheses.

In 1996, magnetic attachments were first introduced outside the country at the Meeting of International College of Prosthodontists, Asia division, and a great attention was paid by the participants. After that, International Research Project of Magnetic Dentistry(IRPMD) was established, and magnetic attachments were widely introduced in the world.

Thus, magnetic attachments are taken notice of their small size, strong retentive force and anti-corrosion in Western as well as Asian countries, and are coming into wide use. Magnetic attachments will bring new possibilities in the field of retention of removable prostheses.

In addition, rapid advancement of industrial technology has produced new type magnet of different materials and structures, and investigations are already started with its applications. Quite new types of magnetic appliances may appear in place of today's magnetic attachments in near future.

Terminology of Magnetic Dentistry

Consistent terminology is important to our ability to communication. The study on the application of magnets on the dentistry started from only three decades ago and current magnetic dentistry has not a long history yet. The terms used in this field have been mostly introduced from magnetic engineering and they are comparatively consistent. However, different terms are used mainly on the original magnetic appliances concerning the concept of their development. The author would like to briefly explain the terms used in this book.

Magnetic attachment is a retentive appliance of dentures using magnet, which belongs to the dental attachment. It consists of the magnetic assembly and the keeper. It is mostly used as a root surface attachment, but used for the retainer of removable bridge or implant as well. Originally, magnetic attachment is the name which was given to the current magnetic appliance in 1980. Before that, magnetic retainer or magnetic appliance was generally used.

Magnetic assembly is a main part of the magnetic attachment which consists of the magnet and the yoke. According to assemblage of these elements, two types are fabricated at the present. Sometimes the magnet is simply used for the magnetic assembly.

Keeper is a metal part of the magnetic attachment which is attracted to the magnetic assembly.

Cup-yoke type or *sandwich-yoke type* indicates the asssemblage of the magnet and the yoke inside the magnetic assembly. Cup-yoke type is such a structure that a cylindrical magnet is set into the cup-shaped yoke, while in the sandwich-yoke type, a cubic magnet is sandwiched in between two cubic yokes, all of which are encapsulated with thin stainless case. *Cap-yoke type* is also used often for cup-yoke type.

Yoke is a metal part inside the magnetic assembly, which is used reinforcement of the attractive force of the magnet according to establishing closed circuit of magnetism.

Closed circuit or *open circuit* of magnetism

explains the flow of the magnetic fulx. In the current magnetic attachment, closed circuit is used, in which the magnetic flux is controlled not so as to spread outside the keeper by the yoke.

Root cap generally means a metal cover of amputated root surface. In magnetic attachment technique, it is used for fixation of the keeper to the abutment root. The keeper is incorporated in casting the root cap or bonded to the root cap by cement or resin. Instead of the root cap, *cast base* or *cast coping* is used sometimes.

Abutment is defined as a tooth used for the support or anchorage of a fixed or removable denture. Actually *abutment tooth* is often used.

Root-keeper system is a unique technique in which the keeper is directly fixed to the root surface with adhesive resin. For that the "root keeper" with a post inserted to the root canal is available. The keeper is fixed by using tooth adhesive self-curing resin and composite resin to the abutment root.

Self-curing resin is a type of resin which polymerizes of itself in normal temperature. It is essential for the fixation of the magnet and the keeper in the magnetic attachment technique. *Autpolymerizing* or *self-polymerizing* is also used for self-curing.

References

1. Drago C J : Tarnish and corrosion with the use of intraoral magnets. J Prosthet Dent, 66: 536–540, 1991.
2. Riley M A, Williams, A J, Speight J D, Walmsley, A D, Harris I R : Investigations into the failure of dental magnets. Int J Prosthontics, 12: 249–254, 1999.
3. Mizutani H, Nakamura K, Ai M : Follow-up study of removable partial denture with magnetic attachment by questionnaire to dentist. J Jpn Prosthodont Soc, 41: 902–909, 1997 (English abstract).
4. Ishihata N, Mizutani H, Ai M : Application of ferro-magnetic alloy for prosthodontics, Part 5. Application of magnetic attachment for prosthodontically hopeless teeth. J Jpn Prosthodont Soc, 31: 1445–1453, 1987 (English abstract).
5. Ishihata N, Mizutani H, Nakamura K, Ishikawa S, Suzuki Y, Ai M : Clinical application making the best use of the properties of the dental magnet. J J Mag Dent, 1: 88–98, 1992 (English abstract).
6. Tsutsui H, Kinouchi Y, Sasaki H, Shiota M, Ushita T: Studies on the Sm-Co magnet as a dental material. J D Res, 58: 1597–1606, 1979.
7. Gillings B R : Magnetic retention for complete and partial overdentures. Part 1. J Prosthet Dent, 45: 484–491, 1981.
8. Gillings B R : Magnetic retention for overdentures. Part 2. J Prosthet. Dent, 49: 607–618, 1983.
9. Okuno O, Ishikawa S, Iimuro F T, Kinouchi Y, Yamada H, Nakano T, Hamanaka H, Ishihata N, Mizutani H, Ai M : Development of sealed cup yoke type dental magnetic attachment. Dent Material J, 10: 172–184, 1991.
10. Tanaka Y, Honkura Y, Arai K, Watarai A, Hiranuma K, Iwama Y : The development of sandwiched-type dental magnetic attachment. J J Mag Dent, 1: 23–29, 1992 (English abstract).

Part 1

Fundamentals of Magnet and Magnetic Attachment

Chapter 2

Magnetic Applications in Clinical Dentistry

Harold W. Preiskel

According to Douglass and Watson[1] unmet prosthodontic needs in the United States are likely to increase during the first half of this century–a pattern that is likely to be reflected in the rest of the developed world. It is not just the needs, but the demands. In combating the ravages of time man, and particularly woman, appear to be taking an ever-increasing interest. While the unrestored loss of anterior teeth is no longer socially acceptable, restoring missing posterior teeth is not so straightforward. Some patients with shortened dental arches appear to function well throughout their lifetimes[2]. Conversely, Oberg et al[3] showed that within the temporomandibular joint there is an increased incidence of disc perforation and bone re-modelling in those without molar support. Since these findings were based on autopsy material it is hard to know what symptoms, if any, were suffered by these individuals. However, Sarita et al[4] showed that as far as patients were concerned only the complete absence of posterior occlusal support, unilaterally of bilaterally, increased the incidence of the risk of developing the signs and symptoms of TMD. Patients aged between 20 and 40 without molar support did show greater degrees of tooth wear. We also know that those whose shortened arches have been restored with removable prostheses do appear to develop increased masticatory forces in chewing over a period of years[5].

If we are to replace the missing teeth are the patients best interests served by a fixed or by a removable prosthsis? The differential degrees of support provided by the mucosa and by the periodontal ligament have taxed the ingenuity of prosthodontists for generations, resulting in some elegant solutions. Similar complications have arisen when a combination of implant and of periodontal support has to be considered. The removable prosthesis, is no less demanding in clinical skills and like its fixed counterparts requires healthy foundations, sound design and meticulous maintenance if a long-lasting result is to be produced[6-8].

Implant prosthodontics has produced a quantum leap in treatment possibilities, and changed our practicing lives, but at a price that is not always measured in monetary terms. There are still times when it is hard to justify invasive procedures such as extensive grafts, and particularly, nerve repositioning techniques carrying significant morbidity risks, to provide support for implants when effective and straightforward alternative procedures are readily available. As for retention, a plethora of effective units is now available for removable prostheses, some with a track record of generations. Meanwhile, the introduction of newer smaller retainers has increased their usefulness.

For a removable prosthesis to be effective it requies to be well-supported, stable, and retentive. One component may contribute to all three factors, but no retainer can be effective in the absence of support or stability. It is not so much the number of Newtons of retention, or grams of force that matter, but the retention characteristics. With a well-supported stable prosthesis, accidental dislodgement can be prevented by a relatively small retentive force. However, this retentive force must build up quickly as soon as the prosthesis begins to move and must operate over a range of at least 300 microns — as no removable prosthesis remains absolutely static in function. This is one reason why laboratory testing, that is so essential to progress, does not provide the full story. Most breakaway forces are tested with very slow separation speeds and with carefully aligned force application. This does not entirely mimic the rapid fire varying force applications that exist in the mouth.

Magnets have demonstrated their usefulness in maxillo-facial prosthodontics and for extra-oral use. It was only the development of rare earth magnets with their high intrinsic coercive forces that allowed size reduction for partial and overdenture retaines. Today, this is the most common application.

Magnetic Retention

There are other important differences in the mechanism of mechanical and magnetic retention systems. At rest, a mechanical retainer may be passive exerting a force only to resist displacement of the prosthesis; a magnetic retainer exerts its maximum retention force when the prosthesis is seated. Magnetic retention forces are vectors with both force and direction components as opposed to temperature which is simply scalar. The force and direction of the magnetic retention varies with position and is known as the magnetic field. The field strengths of magnets employed intraorally are well within generally accepted safety standards.

Some of the earlier magnetic retention systems offered effective retention only when the two components were precisely aligned. A separation of 100 microns reduced the retention to almost zero, clearly an inadequate system for use in the mouth. Furthermore, laboratory testing did not always show up problems of corrosion that plagued so much of the earlier applications of magnets in dentistry. While many of the earlier drawbacks with magnetic retention systems have been overcome, the principles have not altered, namely that maximum retentions is obtained with the component touching and closely aligned and that the retention falls off rapidly with separation. Furthermore, magnetic retention units have very limited resistance to sheering loads. These principles must be understood if these retainers are to be used to maximum advantage.

Multiple retainers do increase retention but not always by very much. The reason is that the prosthesis seldom, if ever, engages all its retention elements simultaneously when subject to a displacing force. However, if the retainers are placed cross arch and widely separated they can add a great deal to the stability of the restoration, together with providing increased support (*Fig 1*).

While the clasp, semi-precious retainer, and precision attachments have given generations of service in removable partial dentures, the overdenture poses somewhat different problems. The key to success is support from the periodontal ligament. However, in an overdenture any structure projecting above the mucosa can only be accommodated by making a corresponding hole in the overdenture. The taller the structure the deeper the hole. Those with some experience in the field know only too well how restricted vertical space can be. There is another drawback with tall root abutments as the higher they are the greater their influence upon the path of insertion of the overdenture — a path that must also take jaw contours into account. Furthermore, those abutments need to be aligned with one another. Even ball and socket attachments have a misalignment tolerance of some 15° if a high rate of

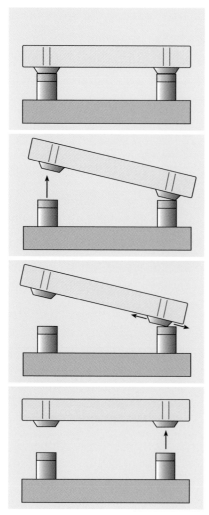

Fig1 Diagrammatic representation to show the separation of a beam retained by two magnets.

wear is to be avoided.

The ideal overdenture retainer will occupy minimal vertical and bucco lingual space, be simple to adjust and maintain while not being unduly technique sensitive. Furthermore, it should be easy to maintain plaque free! Small wonder that few units actually combine all these features.

The magnetic overdenture abutment has a flat surface with little, if any, demands upon the path of insertion of the denture. Being flat it should be readily cleansable. (Fig2,3) Elderly or arthritic patients will not need to struggle in their efforts to find a path of insertion, as the restoration is almost self-seating. As for alignment of the root surfaces, the magnetic keepers do not have to be coplanar simplifying matters still further. Once

the spectre of corrosion has been overcome, and this may well be the case already, we can now concentrate on conventional retention complications such as ensuring that the magnet does not rotate or loosen within the denture base and that the keeper does not rotate or break away from the root or implant.

In implant prosthedontics it took just a few years before the versatility of the removable restoration became appreciated. No longer was artificial tooth position completely dominated by implant position and alignment. The overdenture allowed for similar and less invasive treatment planning with considerable cost advantages as well.

Compared with the root supported restoration the implant retainer is more straightforward requiring no cementation — merely screwing on the appropriate abutment/keeper combination and ensuring that it does not loosen. It is certainly the approach to consider when only minimal abutments are feasible and we await the longer-term treatment outcomes with interest (Fig4).

Clinical Techniques for Magnets

Magnets are straightforward to use in the mouth. As with attachments the location of the magnets within the denture may be carried out in the laboratory or intraorally using the well tried pick up technique. It is largely a matter of operator preference as the Curie temperature of the magnets (the temperature at which it loses its magnetic properties) is above that reached with autopolymerizing acrylic resin. Most magnets begin to lose their attractive force around 150°C so that acrylic resin polymerisation in a microwave with the magnet in place should not be undertaken. This should be remembered when repairs or rebasing are undertaken. A useful aid is a spacer that corresponds with the contours of the magnet. In fact, the spacer should be slightly larger. The denture is waxed up around the spacer so

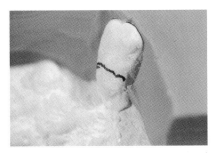

Fig 2 Silicone mould over proposed abutment showing outline preparation.

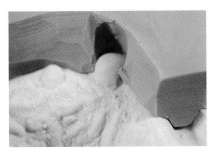

Fig 3 Prepared master cast demonstrating space available for magnetic assembly.

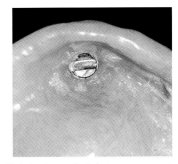

Fig 4 Original sandwich type magnet used as a transitional retainer.

that the amount of space available is clearly seen. Once the trial insertion has been approved the magnet is incorporated before curing the acrylic resin.

A spacer in also useful for intra oral location as nothing is more frustrating than trying to grind a hole in a finished denture and finding insufficient space or perforating the facial aspect of an artificial tooth. With intraoral location it is essential to position the denture in its correct spatial relationship with the abutments and the mucosa. This is relatively straightforward for a partial denture with an occlusal rest as a stop. An overdenture has no such visible positioning device and requires careful seating and checking.

Next, the magnet has to be correctly seated on its keeper ensuring that it is not dislodged as the denture is seated over it. Finally, the two have to be united taking care that no excess resin flows into an undercut locking the entire restoration in place. In practice, a small window should be cut through the denture so that the magnet can be clearly seen through it when the denture is positioned. A small amount of autopolymerizing acrylic resin is inserted through the window to unite the magnet to the denture. Once the magnet has been located, the spaces around it can be filled in with small additions of autopolymerizing resin. For magnets without a plastic cover, an initial placement of resin can be made to ensure that there is good union between denture and magnet.

Where teeth are broken down and a smooth root contour cannot be produced the magnetic keeper can be incorporated in a precious metal casting. The post-retained coping is waxed up in the conventional manner with the root keeper within it. The alignment of the keeper should be parallel with the occlusal plane, if possible, to provide the most effective retention. The magnet can be located within the denture in the laboratory or using a chair side technique.

Chair Side Magnetic Attachment Assembly

The magnetic attachment unit eliminates laboratory procedures and may be accomplished at the chair side. If you are converting a partial denture to an overdenture make sure adequate space is left internal to the ridge lap of the new artificial tooth. The assembly is divided into three stages:

1. Root keeper installation.
2. Implant abutment connection.
3. Location of the magnet within the denture.

Root Keeper Installation

Preparation for the root keeper is critical to the success of the procedure. The miniature magnets occupy minimal vertical space but care must be taken not to interfere with the vertical dimension. Space is a precious commodity. The root surface should therefore be reduced so that the margins are some 2mm supra gingival to allow for periodontal health, but the center of the tooth can be hollowed out. Maximum retention is obtained when the keeper can be positioned at right angles to the displacing forces.

a) Reaming the canal

The keeper post has a length of 7mm. Reaming should be carried out in stages starting with a self-centering device such as a Gates Gidden to establish the length, and then widening the canal in stages. The operator may choose to taper or shorten the post according to the root anatomy.

b) Trial insertion of the keeper

The root face can now be prepared to accommodate the keeper and the trial insertion carried out. If a root facer is available this aids obtaining well-adapted surfaces for the keeper. When satisfactory, the magnet should be placed over the uncemented keeper and the denture placed over it to ensure adequate space has been provided for the assembly. Cutting a lingual or palatal window to allow the magnet to be seen through the denture is helpful. If additional space is needed and cannot be found within the denture further preparation of the root will be necessary.

c) Cementation of the keeper

Remove the keeper, wash and dry the canal. The use of glass ionomer cement or luting composite resin is recommended. The material should be placed in the canal using a spiral filler and the post coated before seating the keeper on to the root face. Ensure that the occlusal surface of the keeper is not scratched when excess material is removed.

If the cement selected requires a metal bonding agent then this agent will need to be applied to the post if any adjustments have to be carried out. The root surface and the canal should be etched for about 20 seconds and then washed with water and dried. The exposed root surface and root canal should be etched with a dentine primer. Use a spiral filler to place resin in the canal, coat the post, and insert the root keeper. Make sure the occlusal surface of the root is smooth taking particular care to protect the occlusal surface of the keeper. You are now ready to proceed with locating the magnet within the denture (*Fig5–7*).

Implant Abutment Connection

Where implants are to be used as abutments the procedure is relatively simple. Today most keeper units are produced with matching abutments. Select the shortest abutment/keeper assembly that will provide a keeper surface about 2 mm above the mucosa. Tighten securely as keeper loosening is a well-documented possible complication.

Magnet Location

Make sure there no undercut surfaces around the root and protect the surrounding mucosa with Vaseline.

Place the magnet over the keeper. Take particular care to ensure that it is the bare surface of the magnet that is placed in contact with the keeper. The resin-covered sections ensure excellent bonding with the denture-base material. The window cut within the denture base should be large enough to allow the denture to be placed over the magnet without dislodging it.

Mix a small amount of autopolymerizing acrylic resin and insert it through the lingual or palatal window over the magnet. Do not attempt to fill the entire void, insert just enough material to connect the magnet to the denture base.

Allow the autopolymerizing resin to cure completely before removing the denture. Ensure that no material has flowed between the magnet and the keeper. Under no circumstances should the keeper surface of the magnet be scratched or damaged. Fill in any void around the magnet with a further mix of self-polymerizing resin and reseat in the mouth. This stage should be carried out in at least two steps taking particular care not to over fill as the additional resin will flow onto the

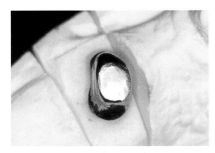

Fig 5 Master cast showing keeper incorporated in the root coping.

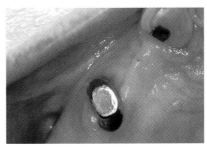

Fig 6 Root coping cemented in the mouth.

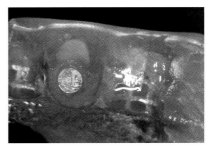

Fig 7 Magnet within the denture.

mucosa or may lodge between the magnet and the keeper. Surplus resin can be removed using a plastic instrument. Never shave or grind the magnet. Do not use very hot instruments in an attempt to remove the magnet from the denture base.

Re check the occlusion. An initial examination with articulating paper ensures that the denture/abutment relationship has not been disturbed. A subsequent check record (remount procedure) is recommended.

Advise the patient to remove the denture when an MRI examination is to be undertaken and inform the patient that there may be some affect on the MRI image due to the keeper. As

with all over denture abutments plaque control and regular maintenance is essential.

It can be seen that the renaissance of magnetic units with 21st Century technology holds considerable promise. We may be making less removable dentures than before, but those that we do construct will need to be made to an exacting standard. Overdentures supported by roots and those supported by implants appear to be gaining in popularity. The removable prosthesis is likely to prove a valuable part of the Prosthodontist's armamentarium for the next two generations in which the newer magnets may well be playing an increasing role.

References

1. Douglas C W, Watson A J : Further nees for fixed and removable partial dentures in the united states. Prosthet Dent, 87(1): 9–14, 2002.

2. Kayser A F: How much reduction of the dental arch is functionally acceptable for the ageing patient? Int dent J, 40: 183–188, 1990.

3. Öberg T, Carlsson G E, Fayers C M : The temporomandibular joint: a morphological study on human autopsy material, Acta Odont Scand, 29: 3, 349, 1971.

4. Sarita P T N, Kreulen C M, Witter D J, Creugers N H J: Sings and symptoms associated with TMD in adults with shortened dental arches. Int J Prosthet, 16(3): 265–270, 2003.

5. Matsumoto M, Sodeyama A, Toda S: A clinical periodical and psychological evaluation of changes in masticato-ry load centre of unilateral shortened arch and those after RPD treatments. J Prosthet Dent, 12(6): 563, 1999.

6. Koivumaa K K: Changes in periodonal tissues and supporting structures connected with partial dentures a clinical histological and roentogenological study, Helsinki Suppl. 52: 172–175, 1956.

7. Kovumaa K K, Hedegard B, Carlsson G E : Studies in Partial Prosthesis 1. An Investigation of Dentogingivally Support Dentures Suomen Hammaslaakariseuran Toimituksia, 56, 1990.

8. Zlatarick D K, Celebic A Valentic, Peruzovic M: The effect of removable partial dentures on periodontal health of abutment and non-abutment teeth. J Periodontol, 73 (2): 137–144, 2002.

The Technology of the Dental Magnetic Attachment

Yoshinobu Honkura

The unique characteristics of the dental magnetic attachment were realized mainly in Europe and America in the 1980's[1-2]. But it failed due to weak retention and corrosion problems. In Japan, a small and highly efficient magnetic attachment, as shown in *Fig1*, was developed through technical progress in recent years. With retentive force per volume increased 10 times over previous products and the corrosion problem solved by laser welding, dental magnetic attachments are now being widely used in Japan and Asia.

In this chapter, the engineering foundation and development progress of the MAGFIT dental magnetic attachment (Aichi Steel, Japan) will be explained focusing on the remarkable improvement in retentive force and solution to the corrosion problem by laser welding[3, 4].

Structure

There are two typical structures for a dental magnetic attachment: a "sandwich-type" and a "cap-type"[5] as shown in *Fig2*[6, 7]. They were comprehensively designed in consideration of size, sufficient retentive force, corrosion prevention, wear resistance and mechanical strength according to requirements for clinical applications. The typical dental magnetic attachment consists of two parts: a magnetic assembly with an internal magnet, and the keeper which is magnetically attracted to the said assembly. The sandwich-type magnetic attachment has a yoke on both sides of the magnet, with a non-magnetic spacer casing in

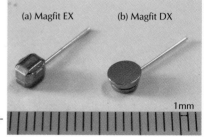

Fig 1 Magfit magnetic attachments.

(a) Magfit EX   (b) Magfit DX

1mm

between them to form part of the magnetic circuit design. These parts are all laser welded together to prevent corrosion. The cap-type magnetic attachment consists of a magnet housed in a cap-shaped yoke which is laser-welded on the bottom to a disc. The laser welded boundary of the disc forms a non-magnetic ring which is an integral part of the magnetic circuit design. The keeper is the same diameter as the magnetic assembly with a thickness of 1mm.

The magnet material is a 358 KJ/m3 class Neodymium Iron Boron (NdFeB) sintered magnet, and the yoke, keeper, and disc parts are manufactured with a soft magnetic stainless steel called AUM20 (Aichi Steel, Japan) with the chemical composition 19Cr-2Mo-0.1Ti. The spacer part casing, ring, and keeper holder are all dental grade non-magnetic stainless steel SUS316 (16Cr-12Ni-2Mo).

The standard retentive force of the magnetic attachment is about 5.9N. With the sandwich-yoke type case, it has an elliptical shape with dimensions of 2.8mm × 3.8mm. The magnetic assembly height is 1.8mm and the keeper height is 1.0mm. For the cap-yoke type, it has a circular

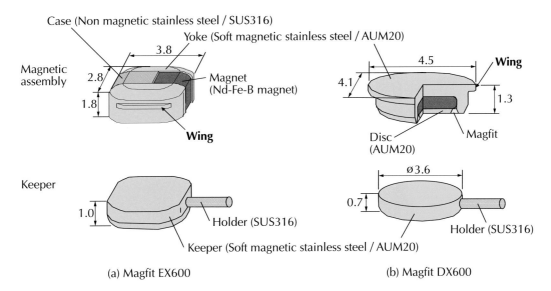

Fig 2　Structure and dimensions.

(a) Magfit EX600

(b) Magfit DX600

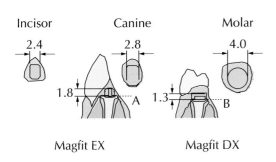

Fig 3　Suitable position of Magfit products.

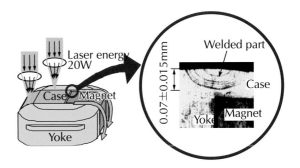

Fig 4　Micro-Laser welding.

shape with a diameter of 3.6mm. The magnetic assembly height is 1.1mm and the keeper height is 0.8mm. In addition to the standard type, there are two other levels of retentive force with 3.9N for the sandwich-type and 3.9N and 7.8N for the cap-yoke type. When looking at the cross-sectional size of all teeth from front teeth to the back molars, and the diameter and height of these teeth, it is possible to apply a magnetic attachment to any size of teeth as shown in *Fig 3*.

The magnetic assembly and keeper are specifically designed to form a closed magnetic circuit to produce maximum retentive force. The engineering concept behind a magnetic circuit is that it should control the line of magnetic flux from the magnet source. This will be explained later, since it is especially important in the design of a magnetic attachment when efficiently converting magnetic energy into retentive force.

In order to protect the internal magnet from corrosion, the outer parts are hermetically sealed together with micro-laser welding, as shown in *Fig 4*. The thickness of the welded parts are only 70μm with a tolerance of ±15μm and exhibit more than sufficient strength. In terms of mechanical endurance, MAGFIT dental magnetic attachments can bear the compression load of 4,413N, as shown in *Fig 5*. Furthermore, there is no measurable decrease in retentive force after a 100,000 cycle load test of 78N. A unique design feature of the cap-yoke type magnetic attachment is that at the time of laser-welding the bottom disc to the cap-yoke type, the melted parts become a non-magnetic component of the magnetic circuit design.

For sandwich-yoke type magnets, small wing-

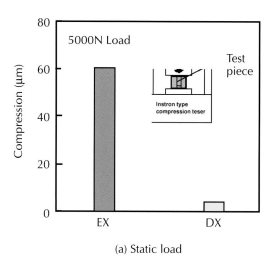

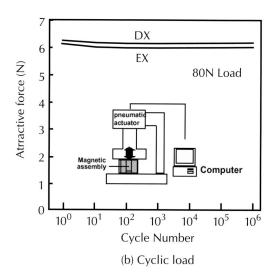

(a) Static load

(b) Cyclic load

Fig5   Mechanical endurance.

type projections are formed on the sides of the yoke. This design feature prevents detachment of the magnet after it is retained with resin in the overdenture. The effect of the wing design is shown in *Fig6*. In addition, a holder, which is used to aid the placement of the keeper before the casting process, is laser welded to the edge of the keeper. The holder has a diameter of only 0.6mm and can be conveniently bent. The hardness of the attractive face of MAGFIT is 200Hv and over the last 10 years, there have been no reports of premature wear or damage of the magnet assembly under normal use. Since magnetic attachments for implant-supported overdentures have high occlusal pressure, a ceramic titanium-nitride (TiN) coating is applied to the attractive face to increase wear prevention.

The Foundation of Magnetic Engineering of the Dental Magnetic Attachment

The basic engineering issues for dental magnetic attachments are:

- The fundamental relationship between the magnet and attractive force
- An effective magnetic circuit design to maximize the use of magnet energy
- Computer-aided optimization of the magnetic circuit design

Based on the above technologies, we can achieve an increase in magnetic attractive force.

What exactly is a Magnet?

In order for someone to understand a magnetic attachment, it is important to understand about the magnet, which is the source of the magnetic force. There are many types of magnets available such as Alnico, ferrite magnets, and rare earth magnets. Since NdFeB has the highest magnet energy among this group, it was chosen for use in the latest dental magnetic attachment and will be explained further.

A magnet has two magnetic poles: a north pole (N) and a south pole (S). These opposite poles are naturally attracted to each other. On the other hand, two of the same poles will oppose each other. This magnetic force acts eternally and permanently. But does it really act eternally? As shown in *Fig7*, a magnet is a collective group of atomic-sized magnets. The electron structure of an atom is shown in *Fig8*. Each electron has an electric charge and "spin" which is the source of magnetic force. Although one pair of electrons exists on the inner orbit near the nucleus and the spin is effectively cancelled, an unpaired electron on the outer shell orbit exists independently, and the spin is preserved which forms an atomic magnet. The Fe atom and Nd atom have unpaired 3d

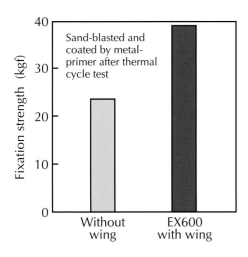

Fig 6 Fixation strength of the magnetic attachments to the denture.

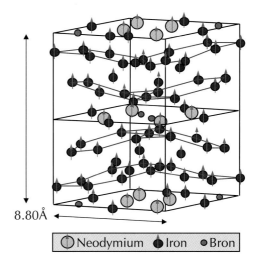

Fig 7 Crystal structure of NdFeB magnet.

electrons and unpaired 4f electrons respectively, and each of them forms an atomic magnet. When these atomic magnet elements Fe and Nd are alloyed at a certain rate, a spin-spin exchange interaction works among these elements, and these atomic magnets are aligned into a specific direction which makes it a magnet of macroscopic size. The magnetic force based on such electron spin acts eternally.

However, the actual magnetic force decreases when exposed to high temperatures or a large external magnetic field. This is because when exposed to these conditions, the orientation of the atomic magnet is disturbed. Furthermore, when chemical composition of the magnet changes due to oxidization, corrosion, etc., or when the magnet physically breaks, the magnetic force is also reduced.

Next, in *Fig 9*, the magnetization characteristics are shown as a B-H curve. In simple terms, a NdFeB alloy can be seen as a container of magnetic energy, but it does not become a magnet until it is induced by a strong, external magnetic field. When an electric current (I) is applied to a coil, it becomes an electromagnet and an external magnetic field is generated. The magnetic strength (H) is calculated by the formula $H=nI/S$ where (n) is the number of coil turns and (S) is the cross-sectional area of the coil. If a strong,

external magnetic field is applied in the opposite direction, the magnetic energy previously held inside the NdFeB alloy will be forced out and, finally will be magnetized in the opposite direction.

Remanent magnetic flux density (Br) and coercivity (bHc) indicate the performance characteristics of a magnet. Br corresponds to the strength of the magnetization of the magnet and bHc stands for the ability to resist an opposite magnetic field. The maximum energy product (BH)max represents the internal magnetic energy of the magnet. Because the attractive force is proportional to (BH)max, it is important to use a magnet with a large (BH)max to get a strong attractive force of the magnetic attachment.

Reference

The strength of a magnetic field (H) and the magnetic flux density (B) have the relationship of $B=\mu H$ (μ is the magnetic permeability of a substance). In a vacuum state, magnetic permeability of the vacuum is expressed as a constant $\mu 0$. In the magnet material, B is the summation of magnetization intensity M ($=xH$), which is made by the alignment of the atomic magnets at a certain direction, and a magnetization intensity of vacuum, $\mu 0H$,. Therefore, $B=M+\mu 0H$ ($=(x+\mu 0)$ H). The magnetization characteristics of the magnet

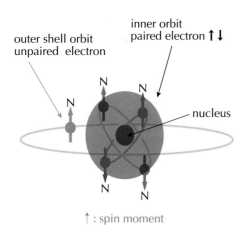

Fig 8   Electronic structure of an atom.

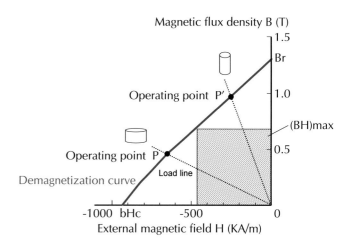

Fig 9   B-H curve and operating point of magnet.

alloy itself is better understood with an M-H magnetization curve (*Fig 10*). However, since the magnet alloy always exists together with the vacuum between atoms, the B-H magnetization curve, which is the sum of both magnetic intensities, is more commonly used.

After magnetization, the magnet itself has an external magnetic field H, whose direction is from the magnetic N pole to S pole, and is opposite to the magnetized direction so that it acts to cancel remananent magnetic flux B as a demagnetizing field. The shorter the magnet, the stronger the demagnetizing field due to the magnetic poles becoming closer together as B is strongly cancelled out. If magnetic shape is decided, the magnetic flux density B and the demagnetizing field H will be determined, and the operating point (P), as shown in *Fig 9*, will be figured out.

Magnets and Magnetic Force

Under Coulomb's Law, the magnetic force (F) is proportional to the strength of the magnetic poles Q_1 and Q_2 and is inversely proportional to the square of distance (r) (Formula1).

$$F=Q_1Q_2/r^2 \quad (1)$$

The magnetic pole strength (Q) is defined as the product of magnetization strength (M), (magnetic strength per unit area), and cross-sectional area (S). Since the magnetization strength

(M) is proportional to the magnetic flux density (B), the magnetic force (F) acting on the material of a cross-sectional area (S) will also be proportional to the square of the magnetic flux density (B) from Formula1.

In order to visualize the magnetic force induced by the magnetic field, a tensioned magnetic flux line is drawn from a magnetic N pole towards the S pole, and the number of the flux lines is proportional to M of the pole. As shown in *Fig 11*, the density of the magnetic flux lines visualizes the strength of the magnetic force of the magnetic material.

Magnetic Circuit

The attractive force of the magnetic attachment is proportional to the square of magnetic flux density (B) at the attractive face and the cross-sectional area (S). A magnetic circuit consists of a magnet, a magnetic material, and a non-magnetic material. Here, the magnet generates the source of the magnetic flux lines which passes through the magnetic material (called a yoke) and hardly passes through the non-magnetic materials. The permeability of magnetic material is about 10,000, and allows many magnetic flux lines to pass through. The magnetic circuit has a similar analogy to an electric circuit as shown in *Fig 12* and can be handled in the same way. One different point from an electric circuit is that in a

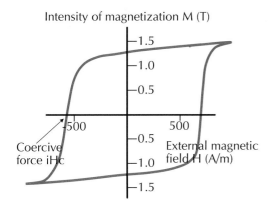

Fig 10 M-H magnetization curve.

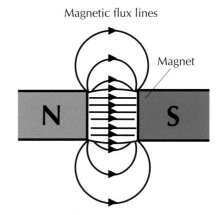

Fig 11 Magnetic field between two magnets.

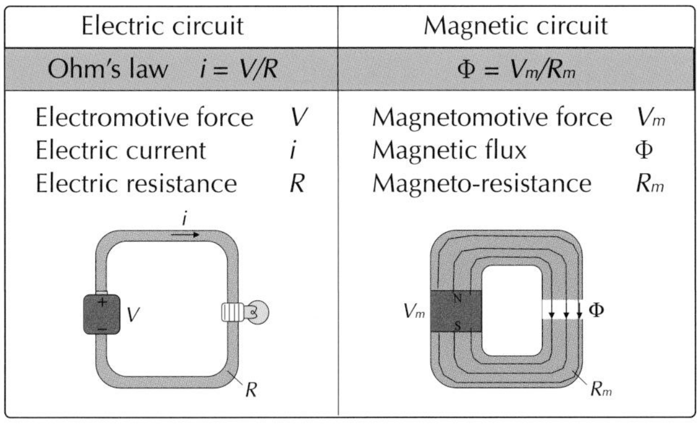

Electric circuit	Magnetic circuit
Ohm's law $i = V/R$	$\Phi = V_m/R_m$
Electromotive force V Electric current i Electric resistance R	Magnetomotive force V_m Magnetic flux Φ Magneto-resistance R_m

Fig 12 Analogy of electric circuit and magnetic circuit.

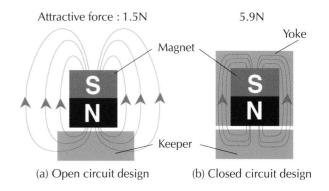

Fig 13 Typical magnetic circuits for magnetic attachments.

magnetic circuit, the magnetic flux line tends to leak from the yoke channel to the outside. This is because the electric resistance of copper wire in an electric circuit is 10^{20} times larger than that of a vacuum, whereas the permeability of magnetic material in a magnetic circuit is just 10,000 times larger than that of a vacuum.

As shown in *Fig 13*, there are two types of magnetic circuits for a magnetic attachment: an open circuit and a closed circuit. The attractive force of a closed magnetic circuit is about four times greater than that of an open magnetic circuit of the same volume. That said, in the case of an open circuit, the magnetic flux lines spread widely all over and the magnetic flux density becomes small at the attractive face. Whereas, in a closed magnetic circuit, magnetic flux lines are concentrated through the attractive face and the magnetic flux density increases. To achieve the maximum attractive force, the magnetic flux density should be equal to the saturation flux density

(Bs) of the entire attractive face. Likewise, when magnetic flux density is maximized, the attractive force is also maximized. Although magnetic flux can be efficiently concentrated through the entire attractive face in the structure of a magnetic circuit, this optimization of the magnetic circuit was very difficult until recent developments in magnetic circuit design.

Computer-aided Optimization of the Magnetic Circuit Design

With the advancement of computer simulation technologies, the optimization of the magnetic circuit made a remarkable improvement of the attractive force in the magnetic attachment[8-9]. The distribution of magnetic flux density (B) is calculated by the finite element method (FEM) based on Maxwell's equations (Formula2, 3) for magnetic fields. The attractive force (F) is calculated by the integration of Maxwell Stress in terms of the entire attractive

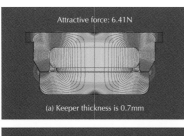

Attractive force: 6.41N

(a) Keeper thickness is 0.7mm

4.20N

(b) Keeper thickness is 0.3mm

Fig 14   Effect of keeper thickness on the attractive force.

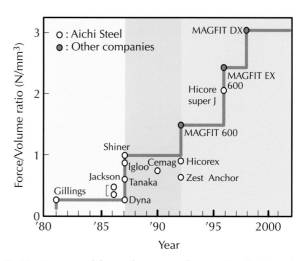

Fig 15   Progress of the performance of magnetic attachment.

face, according to Formula4.

$$(1/\mu) \ \text{rot} \ B = (J + \text{rot} \ M) \qquad (2)$$

$$B = \text{rot} \ A \qquad (3)$$

$$F = (1/\mu) \int (1/2) B^2 (2\cos^2 \vartheta - 1) d\Gamma \qquad (4)$$

The determination of the optimization of the magnetic circuit design are shown in the results of the effect of different keeper thickness on attractive force (*Fig 14*). When a keeper's thickness is optimized, the magnetic flux density (B) is almost equal to the value of the saturation magnetic flux density (Bs) of a magnetic material. On the other hand, if the keeper is too thin, at around 0.3mm, the channel for the magnetic flux lines is not sufficient to let them flow easily and magnetic flux leakage will occur. Therefore, magnetic flux density (B) on the attractive face will decrease from (Bs) and the attractive force will also decrease. In terms of the diagnosis of the magnetic circuit, it is important to achieve the maximum magnetic flux density and saturation magnetic flux density (Bs), and prevent magnetic flux leakage outside the channel.

The Attractive Force Properties of Magnetic Attachments

Since 1981, when Prof. B. Gillings developed the first magnetic retainer, improving the attractive force has been the most important issue. The progress of improvement in attractive force per volume is shown in *Fig 15*. In the last 20 years, there has been about 10 times improvement in attractive force per volume performance, and presently, a small, sufficient magnetic attachment has been successfully developed.

The Challenges of Improving Attractive Force

a) Computer-aided optimization of the magnetic circuit

The optimization of the magnetic circuit made a great contribution to improving the attractive force performance[10, 11]. The effects of various aspects of the magnetic circuit on attractive force using computer simulation are shown in *Fig 16*. *Fig 16a* shows the effect of magnet maximum energy product on attractive force. Although, the increase in attractive force is proportional to the amount of BHmax, it is observed that saturation occurs beyond a certain value. This is because in a specific magnetic circuit design, the maximum number of magnetic flux lines in the channel is already determined for a certain attractive face area and cannot go beyond this set value. The effect of the saturation magnetic flux density (Bs) of a magnetic material on attractive force is shown in *Fig 16b*. Although the attractive force theoretically increases in proportion to the square of Bs, it is actually linearly

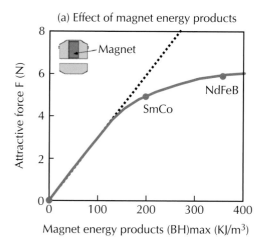

(a) Effect of magnet energy products

Attractive force F (N)

Magnet energy products (BH)max (KJ/m³)

SmCo

NdFeB

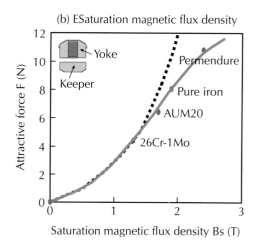

(b) ESaturation magnetic flux density

Attractive force F (N)

Yoke

Keeper

Permendure

Pure iron

AUM20

26Cr-1Mo

Saturation magnetic flux density Bs (T)

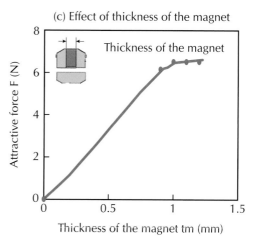

(c) Effect of thickness of the magnet

Attractive force F (N)

Thickness of the magnet

Thickness of the magnet tm (mm)

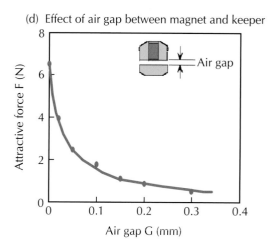

(d) Effect of air gap between magnet and keeper

Attractive force F (N)

Air gap

Air gap G (mm)

Fig 16   Effects of various factors on attractive force.

proportional to (Bs) because of the limits of magnet energy even if saturation magnetic density increases. The effect of keeper thickness as magnetic resistance on attractive force is shown in *Fig 16c*. A keeper is clinically desired to be as thin as possible. However, if it is thinner than a certain value, the attractive force suddenly decreases. This is because the magnetic resistance in the magnetic circuit increases. If an air gap between the magnet and keeper appears, the magnetic resistance increases remarkably and the number of magnetic flux lines decreases as shown in *Fig 16d*. Finally, the effect of the width of laser-welded non-magnetic parts is shown. If the non-magnetic laser-welded parts of Magfit DX become magnetic, a part of the magnetic circuit will short, and magnetic flux lines will flow to other unintended parts and the magnetic flux

density will suddenly decrease and the attractive force is also reduced by half from 5.8N to 2.7N.

It is almost impossible to practically observe each effect of magnet, magnetic materials, and size independently because these factors have intricate and interdependent effects on the attractive force. Therefore, computer-aided analysis made it possible to optimize the magnetic circuit and a much improved, practical magnetic attachment was developed.

b) The significant progress of the magnet

As shown in *Fig 17*, the significant progress of magnet material is remarkable. As previously mentioned, the magnet performance is indicated by maximum energy product ([BH] max) which is proportional to attractive force. Since the discovery of SmCo5 rare earth magnets in 1973,

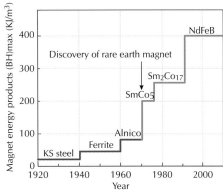

Fig 17 Progress of magnet energy products.

Table 1 Chemical composition of AUM20.

	C	Si	Mn	P	S	Cr	Mo	Ti	Fe
Standard	$\leqq$ 0.020	$\leqq$ 0.50	$\leqq$ 0.40	$\leqq$ 0.40	$\leqq$ 0.005	18.75 / 19.50	1.75 / 2.25	0.10 / 0.30	Balance
Representing value	0.010	0.01	0.02	0.003	0.003	18.9	2.1	0.20	Balance

(Figures in weight %)

magnetic attachments have been able to achieve a practical level of attractive force. With the subsequent invention of higher performance Sm_2Co_{17} and NdFeB magnets[12], the $400KJ/^3$ class magnet came to be used in present magnetic attachments.

c) The development of soft magnetic stainless steel for dental applications

The development of the magnetic stainless steel AUM20 which improved the magnetic characteristics was also important in the improvement of the magnetic dental attachment. The chemical composition of AUM20 is shown in Table 1. Although the Co alloy Permendure, and pure iron have excellent saturation flux density (Bs), they have poor corrosion resistance and cannot be used as a yoke material. While 26Cr-1Mo stainless steel was known as a dental magnetic stainless steel, it did not have the desired magnetic properties. AUM20 was developed by optimizing the chemical composition of Cr, Mo, and Ti while reducing impurities such as C, N, Si, and Mn.

The Debate of Magnetic Circuit Structure: Cap-yoke type or Sandwich-yoke type?

The magnetic circuit structure should be selected before optimizing the circuit. Among numerous magnetic circuit structures which were proposed, two basic designs were focused on[17]. The optimization of the design of both types of magnetic circuit structures progressed and the development of a powerful magnetic attachment was achieved. The relationship of the height and magnet energy product ([BH] max), are shown in Fig 18. When compared with the same cross-sectional area, when the height is as small as 1mm, the cap-type magnetic attachment has a higher attractive force, whereas when the height is higher than 2mm, the sandwich-yoke type magnetic attachment as a higher attractive force. In consideration of the clinical demand for a magnetic attachment, a cap-yoke type magnetic attachment is advantageous when it is applied to the molar region in which the cross-sectional area is large and a thin shape is required. However, when the cross-sectional area is conversely small, but a higher magnetic attachment height is allowed, the sandwich-type is suitable for the front teeth cases.

The Attractive Force Properties of the Magnetic Attachment

The attractive force of magnetic attachments commercially available today range from 3.9N to 10.8N. The bigger the size, the stronger the attractive force. In practical use, some air gap or misalignment between the magnetic assembly and the keeper may appear which may cause a decrease in the predetermined attractive force. If an air gap occurs, the attractive force is drastically reduced as previously shown in Fig 16. Also, when misalignment occurs, as shown in Fig 19,

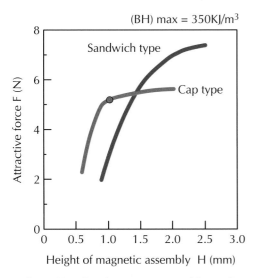

Fig 18 Effect of height of magnetic assembly on the attractive force.

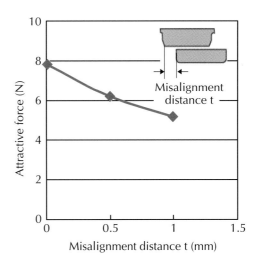

Fig 19 Misalignment distance on the attractive force.

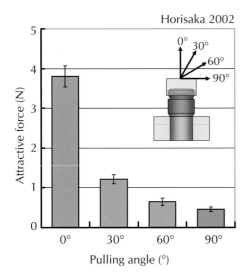

Fig 20 Effect of pulling angle on the attractive force.

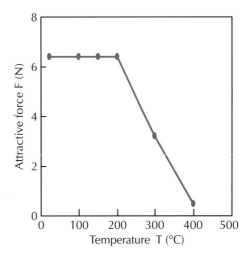

Fig 21 Effect of temperature on the attractive force.

attractive force will decrease. As the attractive face inclines, as shown in *Fig 20*, attractive force decreases with the amount of inclination.

The attractive force originating from the magnet is theoretically eternal. Even if breakaway cycles are repeated, there is no decrease in attractive force. However, the magnet itself will be affected by extreme conditions such as high temperatures beyond Curie point, magnetic corrosion, and strong external magnetic fields which may decrease the attractive force. The effect of temperature on attractive force is shown in *Fig 21*, where demagnetization occurs over 200 degrees C and magnetic force disappears at over 400 degrees C

or Curie points. The effect of a strong, reverse magnetic field is shown in *Fig 22*. With the increase in reverse magnetic field, attractive force decreases gradually and is almost lost at levels more than 1.5T. Next, the influence of corrosion on the magnet due to damage of the magnetic assembly is shown in *Fig 23*. With passage of time in a corrosive environment, corrosion of the damaged magnetic assembly advances, and attractive force is gradually lost up until about 12 months at which point there is no remaining attractive force. Furthermore, self-resilience of attractive force is a big advantage for magnetic retention.

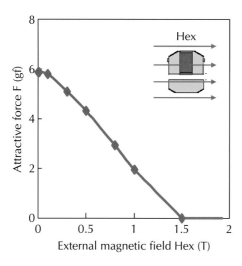

Fig 22 Effect of the external magnetic filed on the attractive force.

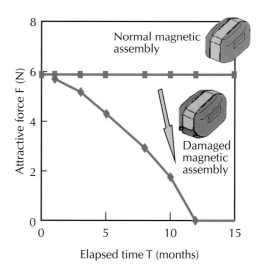

Fig 23 Durability of the attractive force.

Corrosion Prevention and Safety of the Magnetic Attachment

Previously developed magnetic attachments in the early 1980's corroded after use in just 2, 3 years and lost the attractive force. Therefore, magnetic attachments generally suffered a bad reputation from the start. Even today, the negative image for the first generation of magnetic attachments still remains. However, the market acceptance and experience in Japan was quite the opposite, with over 1.2 million units of MAG-FIT magnetic attachments put into clinical use since 1992. The reason for this is that the vastly improved second generation of magnetic attachments did not have the corrosion problem and were widely accepted and used in the dental field.

Corrosion Prevention of Magnetic Assembly

The most important issue is to prevent the corrosion of the magnet. So far, various kinds of preventive measures have been carried out as shown in *Fig24*. The first failed approaches were to simply paint the surface of the magnet with resin, or solder the boundary between a stainless steel casing and magnet. Finally, micro-laser welding of the boundary between a corrosion-resistant stainless steel casing and magnet solved the problem.

The laser welded part, which is shown in *Fig4*, has a sufficient depth of 70µm +15µm to prevent corrosion problem in oralcavity. The liquid penetrant test (JIS Z 2243) is conducted to all the products as shown in *Fig25*, in order to assure the quality of the welded parts. With regards the depth of the welded parts, if it is less than 30µm or less, there is a tendency for the welded seal to break during use. However, as shown in *Fig26*, in order to assure the safety and quality of magnetic attachments, the depth of the welded parts have at least 40µm of depth or more.

Since magnetic stainless steel AUM20 is to be used directly in the oral cavity, excellent corrosion resistance is necessary. As a target, AUM20 was to have corrosion resistance properties superior to previously established dental grade stainless steels such as SUS304 and SUS316[13]. The corrosion phenomenon is the simultaneous electrochemical reaction in which metal ionizes and begins to melt, called an oxidative reaction (at the anode pole) and a deoxidative reaction in which hydrogen ions transforms into hydrogen gas at cathode pole.

There are two types of materials with excellent corrosion resistance: precious metals, such as gold and platinum, which both have a small ionization tendency, and metals with a passive layer

Year	1980~	1987~	1992~
Method	Paint	Soldering /Cementing	Laser Welding
Cap type			
Snad- wich			
Result	Magnet corrosion	Magnet corrosion	No corrosion

Fig 24 Magnet casing sealing methods.

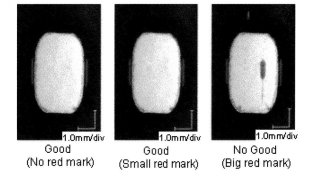

Good
(No red mark) Good
(Small red mark) No Good
(Big red mark)

Fig 25 Liquid penetrant test (JIS Z 2243)

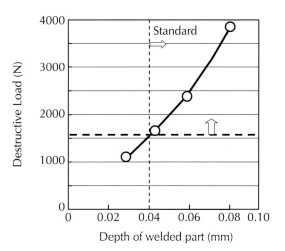

Fig 26 Strength of welded parts.

such as stainless steel and titanium. The corrosion of stainless steel comes in various forms, such as complete corrosion subjected to the outside environment, which often occurs with precious metals, and local corrosion such as pitting corrosion, crevice corrosion, and inter-granular corrosion which occurs when the passive layer is locally destroyed. In consideration of these corrosion forms, some corrosion examining methods are defined by JIS (Japanese Industrial Standards). The results of various JIS examinations of AUM20 and the welded parts between AUM20 and SUS316 are compared with SUS304 and SUS316, as shown in Fig27–29.

As the graph shows, AUM20 and the welded parts between AUM20 and SUS316, has superior results when compared to SUS304 and it has excellent corrosion resistance equivalent to SUS316. Furthermore, the examination result

for artificial saliva in a simulated oral environment are shown in Table 2. The results show that there is no rust and there should be no corrosion problems during regular use in the oral environment[14].

The Corrosion Resistance of the Keeper

The corrosion problem of the keeper is strongly connected to the casting process of the root cap with the keeper. As shown in Fig30, the keeper with root post was originally adhered to the abutment tooth with resin but this method suffered from dental caries problems. Another method, in which a magnetic alloy root cap was cast as the keeper, and then cemented to the abutment tooth was proposed. This method solved the caries problem but retention was insufficient due to the poor magnetic properties of the casting alloy. Since 1992, the newest and

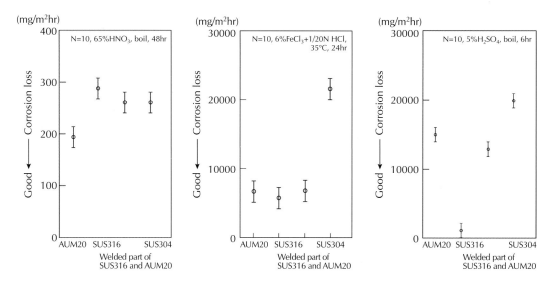

Fig 27 JIS Immersion Test.

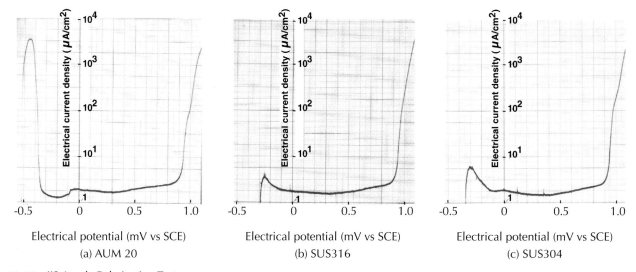

Electrical potential (mV vs SCE)
(a) AUM 20

Electrical potential (mV vs SCE)
(b) SUS316

Electrical potential (mV vs SCE)
(c) SUS304

Fig 28 JIS Anode Polarization Test.

current method was developed to solve both previous problems. The root cap is cast with an incorporated keeper which already has good magnetic properties, and cemented into the abutment tooth.

Current issues which need to be addressed are:

The oxidization problem of the keeper and the resulting crevice corrosion problems between the keeper and the root cap and galvanic corrosion problem between the keeper and root cap alloy.

In order to solve the oxidization and crevice corrosion problems, a Cr rich layer of 15μm was applied to the surface of the keeper as shown in *Fig 31*. And the thickness of the oxidization layer between the keeper and root cap after the casting process is shown in *Fig 32*. As shown, the oxidization layer is very thin and can be removed easily. The results for pit due to crevice corrosion of the laser welded part is shown in *Fig 33*, in which AUM20 with a Cr-rich layer has the lowest amount of pit.

Galvanic corrosion may become a problem between various casting alloys and the magnetic stainless steel AUM20. Furthermore, there is concern that galvanic corrosion may also occur

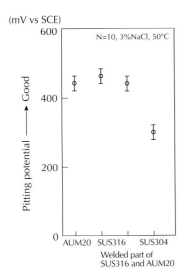

(mV vs SCE)

N=10, 3%NaCl, 50°C

Pitting potential ——→ Good

AUM20 SUS316 SUS304
Welded part of
SUS316 and AUM20

Fig 29   JIS Pitting corrosion potential test.

Table 2   Artificial saliva test of MAGFIT DX600.

Sample No.	Change in appearance	Weight (g)		
		befor test	after test	change
1	none	0.1230	0.1230	0.0000
2	none	0.1229	0.1229	0.0000
3	none	0.1219	0.1219	0.0000
4	none	0.1236	0.1236	0.0000
5	none	0.1222	0.1222	0.0000
6	none	0.1231	0.1231	0.0000
7	none	0.1241	0.1241	0.0000
8	none	0.1226	0.1226	0.0000
9	none	0.1216	0.1216	0.0000
10	none	0.1225	0.1225	0.0000
average		0.12275	0.12275	0.00000

Year	1980~	1987~	1992~
Method	Caries Preformed Keeper	Low retention Cast Keeper	Incorporated Keeper
Material	26Cr-1Mo Stainless steel	Pt-Co-Ni	19Cr-2Mo-0.2Ti Stainless steel
Result	Cause caries	Low retention	No Caries enough retention

Fig 30   Keeper fixation method.

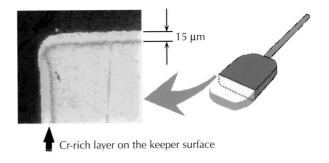

15 μm

↑ Cr-rich layer on the keeper surface

Fig 31   Cross-sectional view of Cr layer.

between Ti implants and AUM20. Thus, these issues were investigated using a potentiometer in Fig 34. Consequently, as shown in Table 3, corrosion current between AUM20 and other metals was very low, so there should be no problems with galvanic corrosion.

Biocompatibility

Biocompatibility tests were conducted on laboratory rabbits as shown in Fig 35. Specimens for the tests were AUM20 laser welded with SUS316 and AUM20 laser welded with Au-Ag-Pd alloy.

Both specimens were directly inserted into the test rabbits. Other specimens were used in elution tests and these eluded solutions were injected into the test rabbits. The following tests were conducted based on the Japan Health, Labor and Welfare Ministry guidelines for Medical Devices: ①Acute toxicity test ②Intracutaneous reaction test ③ Pyrogen test ④Hemolytic test ⑤Implant test. All tests were passed and showed no abnormal results[22].

In terms of nickel allergies, there have been no reports that this is a problem among many clinical treatments carried out in Japan. As dental grade stainless steel SUS316 already in use contains 12% nickel, it cannot be fully declared that nickel does not elude nor cause nickel allergies. To address the potential nickel allergy issue, some magnetic attachment products are applied with a Ti coating or special TiN coating as a special feature.

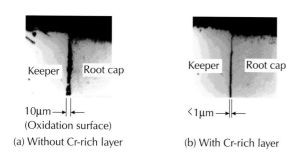

(a) Without Cr-rich layer   (b) With Cr-rich layer

Fig 32   Oxidization reduction with Cr layer.

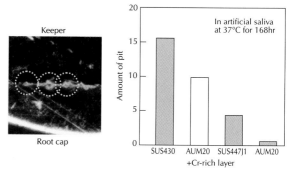

(a) The appearance of pit (AUM20)   (b) Amount of pit in different stainless steel parts

Fig 33   Corrosion pit on the welded parts.

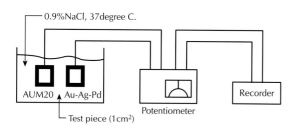

Fig 34   Galvanic corrosion test setup.

Table 3   Galvanic corrosion test results.

Combination		Current (nA/cm²)	Evaluation
Cathode	Anode		
Au-Ag-Pd	AUM20	80	Excellent
Au-Pt	AUM20	80	Excellent
Ag	AUM20	90	Excellent
AUM20	Ti	90	Excellent
AUM20	AUM20	60	Excellent
Ti	Ti	100	Excellent

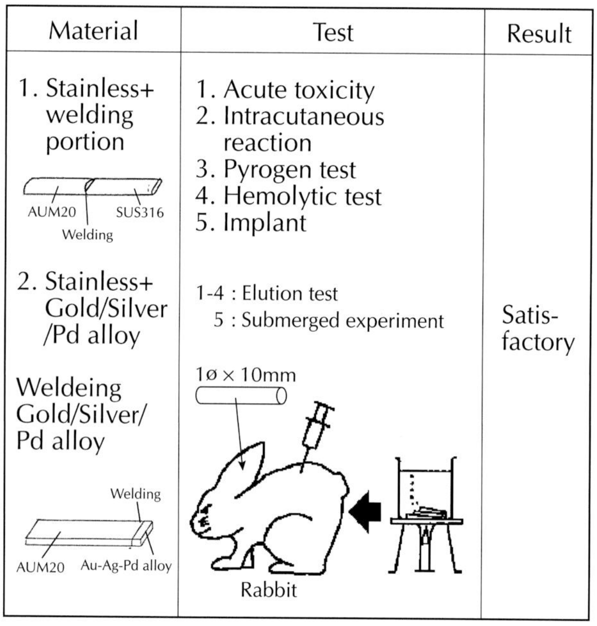

Different metals (rows 1–4), Same metal (rows 5–6)

Material	Test	Result
1. Stainless+ welding portion AUM20 — SUS316 Welding	1. Acute toxicity 2. Intracutaneous reaction 3. Pyrogen test 4. Hemolytic test 5. Implant	Satisfactory
2. Stainless+ Gold/Silver /Pd alloy Weldeing Gold/Silver/ Pd alloy AUM20 — Au-Ag-Pd alloy Welding	1-4 : Elution test 5 : Submerged experiment 1ø × 10mm Rabbit	

Fig 35   Animal Biocompatibility Test.

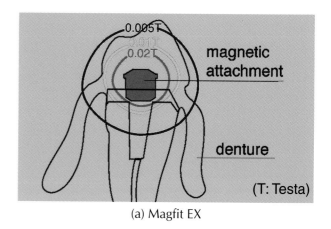

(a) Magfit EX

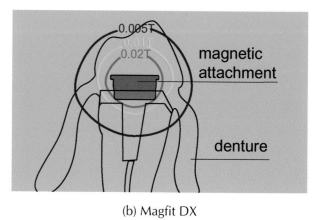

(b) Magfit DX

Fig 36   Magnetic flux leakage.

The Concerns of Magnetic Leakage Flux

As open circuit type magnetic attachments have a relatively large magnetic flux leakage of 0.3T, there is concern about this affecting the human body. However, because of the closed magnetic circuit design, Magfit EX and DX magnetic attachments have a very small magnetic flux leakage of only 0.01T at a 1mm perimeter distance from the attractive surface as shown in *Fig 36*. This level of magnetic flux leakage seems to be not a problem because it is less than the provisional U.S. Safety Standard of 0.02T[15].

References

1. Andrew Paul L H Dias: Retentive Prostheses with Magnets, Proceedings of the Symposium on Magnetic Attachment System. Hong Kong, Hong Kong Prosth Dent Soc, 1998.
2. Tsutsui H: The application of Sm-Co magnet for dental field. Japan, DMA Research Group, 1983.
3. Tanaka Y: Dental Magnetic Attachment. Tokyo, Ishiyaku, 1992.
4. Honkura Y: Progress of Magnetic Applications in the Dental Field J Mag in Jpn, 26(1): 13-17, 2002.
5. Ai M: Removable Partial Dentures Using Magnetic Attachments. Tokyo, Quintessence, 1994.
6. Tian L, Watarai A, Arai K, Honkura Y: Development of a Thin Dental Magnetic Attachment with a Capped Magnetic Circuit. J Mag in Jpn, 23 (4-2): 1573-1576, 1999.
7. Ai M, Hiranuma K: Clinical Application of Magnetic Attachments. Tokyo, Quintessence, 2000.
8. Tanaka T, Satoh A, Kawase J: Design and Application of AC Electromagnets. Tokyo, Morikita, 1991.
9. Kawase J, Yoshida T, Yamaguchi T: Institute of Electrical Engineers Static・Revolving Devices Joint Research Group Data. SA–92–34, RM–92–69: 143, 1992.
10. Honkura Y, Tanaka Y, Iwama Y: Development of Dental Magnetic Attachment with Rare Earth Magnet. J Mag in Jpn, 14(2): 477-482, 1990.
11. Honkura Y, Tian L, Watarai A: Size Perfomance of the Attractive Force for a Dental Magnetic Attachment. J Mag in Jpn, 20(2): 693-696, 1996.
12. Tanaka Y, Hiranuma K, Iwama Y and Honkura Y: Sealed Dental Magnetic Attachment Developed by Three-Dimensional Magnetic Analysis. Proc. 10th Int. Workshop on Rare Earth Magnet and Their Application: 147-156, 1988.
13. Takada Y, Okuno O: Corrosion Behavior of Stainless Steels and Dental Precious Alloys Used for Dental Magnetic Attachments. J Jpn Soc Mag Dent, 3(1): 14-22, 1994.
14. Honkura Y: Soft Magnetic Stainless Steel Materials Research, dissertation. Nagoya, Nagoya University, 1991.
15. Shiga K, Miyamoto H, Ueno T: Effect of Magnetic Fields on Living Organisms. Tokyo, Terapeiya, 1991.

Chapter 4

Biological Effects of Magnetic Attachments on the Human Body and Tissues

Tetsuo Ichikawa／Naeko Kawamoto

Introduction

In recent years, many researchers and clinicians have investigated magnetic and electromagnetic devices for medical and dental uses, such as MRI and magnetic dental attachment. With increased urbanization and prevalence of electromagnetic appliances is common use in daily life, we are subjected to frequent exposure to electromagnetic fields of various frequencies and the biological hazard has also been pointed out[1].

In the prosthodontic field, magnetic attachment that helps to retain overdenture is being widely used in Japan and becomes popular in Asian region[2]. In addition, these devices have been used for dental implants. But there are few data in the literature on the effects on bone tissue of a static magnetic field created by a magnetic dental attachment

In this paper we review the biological effect of electromagnetic fields, in particular a static magnetic field, showing the results of *in vitro* and *in vivo* experiments.

Classification of Electromagnetic Field and Biological Effects

Electromagnetic fields are categorized into two: static magnetic and alternative magnetic fields. Alternating magnetic fields, which have changes of intensity over time, range from extremely low frequency (ELF, $30 \sim 300Hz$) produced by consumer electronics, to the ultra high frequency (UHF, $300MHz \sim 3GHz$) produced by

mobile phones and microwave ovens, and also include cosmic rays. Static magnetic fields with an intensity that is almost invariant with time, also include the magnetic fields of the earth (50-100μT, T:Tesla), as well as those of MRI (1.5-2.0 T), and magnetic attachments (0.4-0.8 T)[3] (*Fig1*).

In alternating electromagnetic fields, it is often suggested that overhead power transmission lines may affect human body harmfully[4]. According to the proposed hypothesis, electromagnetic field exposure has the ability to potentiate or amplify cell signaling[5]. Although extensive research on these electromagnetic fields has been performed, experimental studies have produced contradictory findings regarding the effects of magnetic fields on the human body and tissues.

In static magnetic fields, there is also extensive research that has produced contradictory results. It is known that erythrocytes, containing paramagnetic hemoglobin and flowing in a model vessel were shown to be attracted towards the stronger magnetic field, when exposed to a non-homogenous magnetic field with a steep gradient[6]. It is also reported that oriented fibrin gels were formed by polymerization in strong magnetic fields[7] and collagen fibers orientated perpendicular to the static magnetic fields[8]. Mutagenetic effects of chronic exposure to static magnetic fields have also been investigated. There were no apparent teratogenic effects when embryos were cultured for 20 hrs from the stage of uncleaved fertilized egg to the neurula stage under strong magnetic fields of 8 T[9]. Drosophila larvae, in contrast, have been reported to show abnormalities in embryogenesis during exposures to static magnetic fields as low as 1 mT[10].

Although the above findings suggest that the effects of magnetic attachments on the human body and tissues are not fully understood, it is a fact that various apparatuses using electromagnetic field are commercially available for personal use.

Biological Effect of Magnet Assembly

Magnetic intensity of a dental attachment (Aichi Steel) is about 0.8 T on the surface of the magnetic assembly. Leakage flux on the magnet assembly is about 0.01-0.03 T under the condition of contact with a keeper, and about 0.005 T beyond the abutment tooth. Although the magnetic attachment is placed in the mouth for a long period, the magnetic field exposure reaches a restricted area. The above findings show that leakage flux is negligible because the flux is contained in a closed magnetic circuit passing the U.S. safety standards for human body of 0.02 T[11].

In vitro experiment

A static magnetic field exposure system was fabricated for an *in vitro* experiment[12]. The static magnetic field was made between an upper and lower magnet disk of 110 mm in diameter. The intensity of the magnetic field was about 20-80 mT. Mouse osteoblastic MC3T3-E1 cells were cultured on specimens (10×10 mm) of pure titanium in a 24-well plastic plate. The plate was placed in the center of the space and exposed to the static magnetic field. After 3 days in culture, cell proliferation was greater than that of the control without exposure to the static magnetic field. After 1 week, when the intensity of magnetic field was about 20 mT, the cells spread over the entire titanium surface and the extracellular matrix was abundant. (*Fig2a–d*).

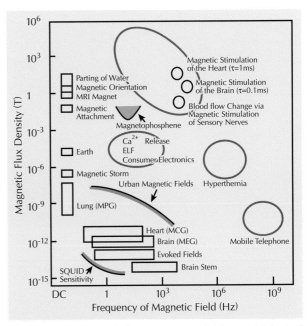

Fig 1 Classification of electromagnetic fields and biological effects. (DC=a static magnetic field). (quotation and revision from Ueno S, Iwasaka M : Biological effects of magnetic and electromagnetic fields. p2, Plenum Press, New York. 1996.).

In vivo experiment

A magnetic disk (4.0 mm in diameter and 1.3 mm in height) sealed by pure titanium was fabricated and the intensity is about 90 mT on the surface. Using rats, inserted the magnetic disk into one femur designated an experimental side and inserted pure titanium disk without a magnet assemble into the contralateral femur as a control group. Rats were sacrificed at 1, 3, and 12 weeks after implantation. We histologically observed the bone-disk interface by light microscopy.

After one week, there was little difference between the two groups. After three weeks, a remarkable difference was observed. Bone tissue with a regular width was observed around the titanium disk in the controls, while various tissues, such as bone marrow, fibrous tissue, and cartilage tissue were observed around the magnetic disk. The magnetic disk was surrounded with abundant new trabecular bone with expanded blood vessels. After 12 weeks, the difference between both groups tended to decrease and new trabecular bone around the magnetic disk tended to be maintained after healing. (*Fig3a–d*).

Fig2a–d In vitro experiment / Cell proliferation and extracellular matrix on Ti disk (bar=10μm)

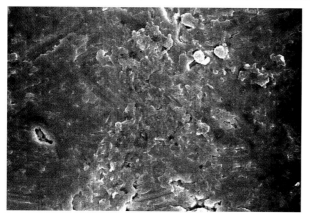

Fig 2a After 3 days under a static magnetic field

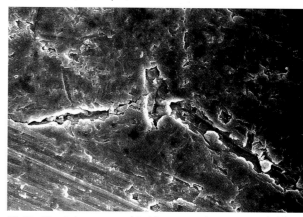

Fig 2b After 3 days control (without a static magnetic field)

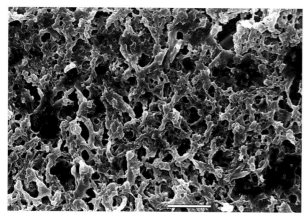

Fig 2c After 1 week under a static magnetic field

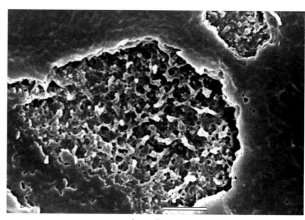

Fig 2d After 1 week control (without a static magnetic field)

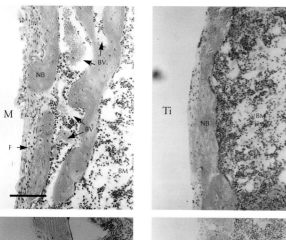

Fig3a–d In vivo experiment / Bone-disk interface (HE stain, bar=100μm).
Ti: pure titanium. M: magnetic assembly sealed in pure titanium. NB: new bone. BM: bone marrow. BV: blood vessel. F: fibrous tissue

a | b

Fig 3a 3w 90mT
Fig 3b 3w control

c | d

Fig 3c 12w 90mT
Fig 3d 12w control

In this study, the magnet was completely sealed by pure titanium using micro-laser technique, and there was no dissolution of magnetic material. Therefore, it is suggested that the static magnetic field greatly influenced bone remodeling of immature tissue greatly during the healing process, but there was little effect on remodeling after healing. Influence of static magnetic fields varies with the intensity and exposure time, phase of cell division.

Summary

We conclude that the static magnetic field induced by a dental magnetic attachment has little effected on the human body and tissues. Our in vitro and in vivo experiments show that magnetic attachments might have an effect on immature bone tissue immediately after implant placement, but the effect may to accelerate the bone remodeling.

References

1. Polk C, Postow E : Handbook of Biological Effects of Electromagnetic Fields (2sd Ed). New York, CRC Press, 1996.
2. Thean H P, Khor S K, Loh P L : Viability of magnetic denture retainers: a 3-year case report. Quintessence Int, Jul–Aug, 32(7): 517–520, 2001.
3. Ueno S, Iwasaka M : Biological effects of magnetic and electromagnetic fields. Edited by Ueno, S. p1, Plenum Press, New York, 1996.
4. Wertheimer N, Leeper E : Electrical wiring configurations and childhood cancer. Am J Epidemiol, 109: 273–284, 1979.
5. Liburdy R P : Calcium signaling in lymphocytes and ELF Fields: Evidence for an electric field metric and a site of interaction involving the calcium ion channel. FEBS Lett, 301: 53–59, 1992.
6. Okazaki M, Maeda N, Shiga T : Effects of an inhomogeneous magnetic field on flowing erythrocytes. Eur Biophys J, 14: 139–145, 1987.
7. Torbet J, Freyssinet J M, Hudry-Clergeon. : Oriented fibrin gels formed by polymerization in strong magnetic fields. Nature, 289: 91–93, 1981.
8. Torbet J, Ronziere M C : Magnetic alignment of collagen during self-assembly. Biochem J, 219: 1057–1059, 1984.
9. Ueno S, Iwasaka M : Early embryonic development of frogs under intense magnetic fields up to 8T. J Appl. Phys. 75 (10): 7165–7167, 1994.
10. Ho M W, Stone T A, Jerman I, Bolton J, Bolton H, Goodwin B C, Saunder P T, Robertson F : Brief exposures to weak static magnetic fields during early embryogenesis cause cuticular pattern abnormalities in Drosophila larvae. Phys Med Biol, 37: 1171–1179, 1992.
11. WHO: Environmental Health Criteria 69 / Magnetic Fields. WHO. Geneva, 128, 1987.

Chapter 5

Influences of Magnetic Attachments on Medical Appliances

Toshio Hosoi∕Fujio Tsuchida

Magnetic attachments in the oral cavity are anticipated to influence medical appliances in some patients. In the clinical setting, magnetic resonance imaging (MRI) and the cardiac pacemaker are thought to be of particular concern. It is important to advise patients of these potential influences before using magnetic attachments in dental treatment. The present paper introduces anticipated influences and solutions to potential problems associated with the use of magnetic attachments.

Influences on MRI

Resonance phenomena occur when an atomic nucleus is placed in a fixed magnetic field and electromagnetic energy of a certain frequency is applied. MRI is based on this principle. Specific electromagnetic waves are directed to the human body in a strong magnetic field. MRI is used broadly and is an important tool (*Fig 1*), for example in cervical diagnosis[1]. Unlike X-ray examination, MRI examination involves no exposure to radiation and offers an excellent resolving power for soft tissues. MRI has been clinically applied not only in the medical field but also in the dental field, especially to mandibular joints (*Fig 2*). Before MRI examination, patients must remove all metal objects from their person in order to avoid the influencing the imaging. Although a denture with magnetic attachments can be removed easily, the magnetic keepers remain in the oral cavity. Magnetic keep-

ers of magnetic stainless steel have a soft magnetic body that is magnetized in a magnetic field but demagnetized outside of a magnetic field. Therefore, MRI is anticipated to cause local image influences.

Actual Example of Influences

Imanaka et al.[2] conducted an experiment to examine artifacts caused by dental materials in MRI. This experiment clarified that Au, Ag, Au-Ag-Pd, and Am contained in general dental filling and prosthetic materials are not influential, whereas Fe, Ni, Cr, and Co contained in base materials do influence imaging. This problem can be solved by removing the denture. However, the question as to whether magnetic keepers for magnetic attachments remaining in the oral cavity might influence imaging. In general, the existence of a magnetic keeper does not affect MRI of frequent brain imaging. But MRI may be affected if disease, such as malignant tumor in the molar soft tissue of the maxilla, is suspected to be present in the oral cavity (*Fig 3a, b*).

Positional Influences

It is important to examine the influences of magnetic attachments on MRI according to the sizes, positions, and number of magnetic keepers. By varying the positions and number of magnetic keepers, Yoshida et al.[3] studied the influences on MRI examination of the brainstem. As the number of magnetic keepers increased, image degra-

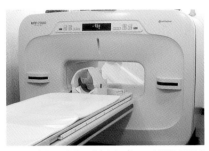

Fig 1 Outline of MRI machine (Hitachi Medico, MRP-7000 0.3 Telsa).

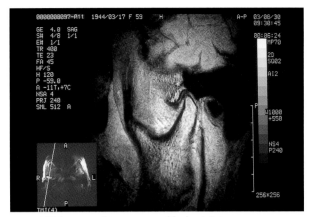

Fig 2 MR images of tempromandibular joint.

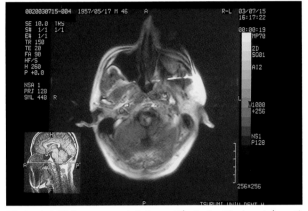

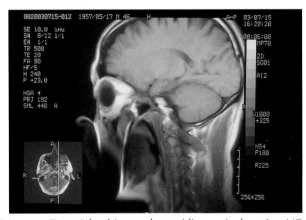

Fig 3a, b MR images containing artifacts (a. Horizontal section MR image, T1 weighted image, b. meridian sagittal section MR image, T1 weighted image). The magnetic keeper was placed on the maxillary left molar. a | b

dation increased. Influences were especially great for the case on which a magnetic keeper was close to the object being imaged. Even when there were no influences on the brainstem, the tongue and palate in the oral cavity showed influences (*Fig4*). Therefore, depending on the position of MRI examination, this may necessitate the removal of magnetic keepers. In contrast, if the doctor or dentist requesting the MRI does not have appropriate knowledge, magnetic keepers may be removed unnecessarily. If the removal of magnetic keepers is requested by a medical institution for the purpose of MRI examination, we must determine whether or not the magnetic keepers should be removed.

Solutions

Even when influences on MRI are anticipated, sealing the magnetic keepers may be difficult, and removing the magnetic keepers may be a

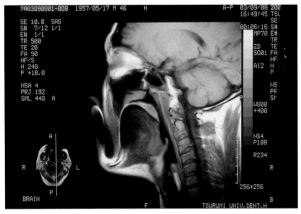

Fig 4 MR images containing artifacts (sagittal section MR image, T1 weighted image). The magnetic keeper was placed on the mandibular left premolar.

more effective means by which to avoid magnetic influences during imagery. It is possible, but not easy, to remove only magnetic keepers from a coping fabricated by casting. Unlike casting, direct bonding method does not involve the application of heat, but rather uses magnetic keepers as they are with priority given to the plane characteristic[4]. Since the coping and mag-

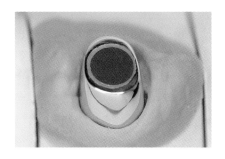 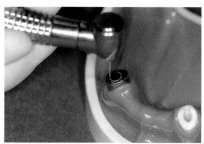

Fig 5 Coping with a keeper is completed by the direct bonding method.
Fig 6 Simulation of magnetic keeper removal using a turbine.

5 | 6

netic keepers are bonded with adhesive resin cement, a clear cement line appears (*Fig 5*) which serves as a guide for removing the magnetic keepers and makes the removal easy (*Fig 6*). The direct bonding method also supports the intraoral method and allows the magnetic keepers to be reattached after MRI examination.

Influences on Pacemaker

Recently available pacemakers are designed so as not to be affected by ordinary magnetic influences. However, some models that are currently in use have a parameter called magnet rate that is affected by magnetism. In an experiment by Miyata et al[5]. using Magfit 600 (Aichi Steel), a magnetic attachment influenced only an SSI-type pacemaker (SIEMENS) when the attachment was placed close to the center of the pacemaker and not when the attachment was moved, even slightly, from this position. Since magnetic bodies are not able to be placed this close to pacemakers in daily life, there may be no magnetic influences.

References

1. Ross J S : Magnetic resonance angiography of the head and neck : A teaching file, St.Louis, Mosby, 1-12, 1994.
2. Imanaka M, Kobayashi K, Yamamoto A : Magnetic resonance imaging artifacts about dental materials. J Jpn Soc Oral and Maxillofac Radiology, 30(3): 33-37, 1990 Japanese.
3. Yoshida M, Furukawa K, Takashima T, Horii Y, Ishibashi K, Itou S, Sakamaki K : Effects of the dental magnetic keeper on MRI - positional distinction, J J Mag Dent, 3(1): 1-8, 1994 (English abstract).
4. Hirano T, Sugiyama K, Mizuno Y, Tsuchida F, Motonaga M, Hosoi T : The laboratory procedure of magnetic attachment by direct bonding method. J J Mag Dent, 12(2): 1-6, 2003 (English abstract).
5. Miyata H, Tanaka Y, Ishigami T, Kishimoto Y, Kiba H, Arai K, Honkura Y : Expeimental Observations of an effect of dental magnetic attachments on a cardiac pacemaker. J J Mag Dent. 2(1): 11-17, 1993 (English abstract).

Chapter 6

The New Generation of Dental Magnetic Attachment

Yoshinobu Honkura

In Japan, a new generation of strong magnetic attachments without corrosion problems called Magfit has been developed and the performance characteristics continue to improve. The results over the last ten years has seen 1.2 million units used widely.

Specifications and Performance of Magfit Magnetic Attachments

The Magfit lineup of products are shown in Table1. They are divided between magnetic attachments for natural tooth root or implant applications. Initially, Magfit for natural tooth root was introduced with five different magnet types with a difference in rigidity. The standard type magnetic attachment has a flat attractive face with two different types: the elliptical-shaped Magfit EX and the round-shaped Magfit DX.

A soft type magnet attachment called Magfit RX has a dome-shaped attractive face with a rotational movement and Magsoft has a cushion function which also has a rotational movement. Furthermore, there is a precision type magnetic attachment with rigid characteristics. Retentive force of the magnet ranges from 3.9N to 7.8N, and the average diameter size of the magnet ranges from 2.8mm to 4.0mm in consideration of the size of the cross-sectional area of abutment teeth. For preparation of root surface, there are three kinds of keepers: the incorporated cast keeper, the removable keeper with screw, and a resin-coping root keeper.

The standard type magnets are Magfit EX and Magfit DX. For Magfit EX, the retentive force range is from 3.9N to 5.9N. The minor axis length is 2.4mm and 2.8mm and is suitable for incisor and canine teeth[1]. For Magfit DX, the retentive force range is from 3.9N to 7.8N. The height of the magnetic assembly ranges from 1.0-1.3mm and since the height is low enough, it is suitable for molars.

The specialty-type magnets are Magfit RX with dome shaped attractive surface, cushion type Magsoft, and precision type Magfit PR as shown in (Fig1). The attractive force of the Magfit RX is 5.9N and this one type can only be used with resin-coping root keeper with convex surface. This convex surface of the keeper and the attractive face of the magnetic assembly are coated with TiN to increase the wear resistance. It is suitable for free-end saddle dentures because the harmful rolling force on the abutment tooth can be reduced. Magsoft has two retentive forces, 4.9N and 7.4N. The cushion cap has the capability for a vertical movement of 0.20mm. And with 6 degrees of rotational function, it can accommodate a wider range of denture movement when compared to Magfit RX. The precision type Magfit PR magnetic attachment has a rigid function from the combination of a sleeve on the magnetic assembly which precisely fits onto a stepped keeper. There are three heights of the step: 0.2mm, 1.0mm and 2.0mm. The retentive force is 3.9N and 7.8N for a total of six different types[5].

Table 1: Magfit magnetic attachments lineup

Intended use	Magnetic assembly			Keeper		Height in total (mm)	Attractive force (N)	Attractive force performance (N/mm³)	Remarks
	Product name	Magnetic structure	Dimensions (mm)	Coping method/ Connecting method	Dimensions (mm)				
Natural tooth	Magfit EX (600)	Closed sandwich	3.8-2.8 × 1.8	Cast	3.8-2.8 × 1.8	2.8	5.9	0.21	Wing
	Magfit DX (600)	Closed cap	ø 4.0 × 1.2	Cast	ø 3.6 × 0.7	1.9	5.9	0.31	Wing
				Root Keeper	ø 3.6 × 0.7	1.9	5.9	0.31	Wing Post: 1.2 × 7
				Removable keeper	ø 3.5 × 2.2	3.4	5.4	0.17	Wing
	Magsoft (S)	Closed cap	ø 4.5 × 1.6	Cast	ø 3.6 × 0.7	2.3	4.9	0.21	Taper Rotation, cushion
				Root Keeper	ø 3.6 × 0.7	2.3	4.9	0.21	
				Removable keeper	ø 3.6 × 2.2	3.8	4.4	0.11	
	Magfit RX	Closed cap	ø 4.4 × 1.4	Root Keeper	ø 4.4 × 1.0	2.2	6.4	0.19	Taper Rotation Post: 1.2 × 7
	Magfit PR (800-2)	Closed cap	ø 5.0 × 3.3	Cast	ø 5.0 × 2.6	3.9	7.8	0.10	Undercut Rigid
Implants	Magfit DX	Closed cap	ø 4.4 × 1.3	Keeper screw	ø 4.7 × 1.4	2.7	7.4	0.18	Wing
	Magsoft	Closed cap	ø 5.2 × 1.8			3.2	6.9	0.10	Taper Rotation, cushion
	Magfit RX	Closed cap	ø 4.4 × 1.4		ø 4.7 × 1.4	2.8	5.9	0.14	Taper Rotation
	Magfit PR	Closed cap	ø 5.0 × 3.2		ø 5.1 × 3.0	4.2	5.9	0.07	Undercut Rigid

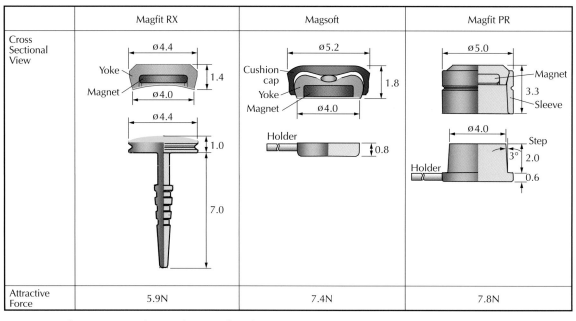

Fig 1 Comparison of magnetic attachments for natural tooth.

The keeper with holder, is meant to be cast into the root cap to form an incorporated keeper. The holder is laser-welded to the side of the keeper in order to stabilize it in the investment material during the casting process, after which the holder is cut off. The removable keeper is intended for easy and convenient removal such as when a patient has to undergo an MRI test. As

shown in (*Fig 2*), the middle plate is cast into the root cap and a screw holds the ring keeper in place. There is already five years or more of clinical experience, and the reliability of the screw part has been evaluated. Using dual curing composite resin, the root keeper is adhered to the tooth root and makes one day treatment possible[3]. Magfit RK has bendable and non-

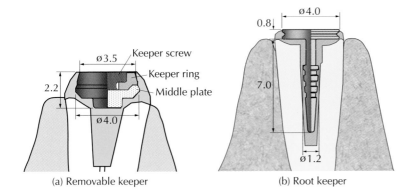

(a) Removable keeper (b) Root keeper

Fig 2 Cross-sectional view of keeper types.

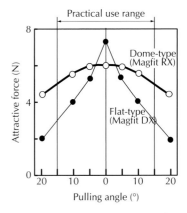

Fig 3 The effect of pulling angle on attractive force of Magfit DX (flat-type) and Magfit RX (dome-type).

bendable type root posts, with the bendable root post neck being able to change the post angle to accommodate different root canals. Since it uses a resin coping, Magfit RK can be used for patients who may need to remove them for MRI tests easily[4].

MAGFIT-IP for Implant Applications

Magfit-IP for implants have 3 types of magnetic attachments: Dome type, cushion type, and flat type[5, 6]. Dome type is suitable for 2-point implant supported overdentures which is free-end saddle dentures. With a dome type magnet, the attractive force of 5.9N may be considered to be a little weak, but as shown in (Fig 3), it is rather stronger than that of a flat type magnet during the rotational movement of the denture. In terms of the wear resistance for dome type magnetic attachment, a TiN coating is applied to the attractive faces to improve its wear resistance. The cushion type magnetic attachment reduces the stress on the abutment implant fixtures with the rotational and cushioning function. It is also recommended for use in 2-point implant supported overdentures. The flat type magnetic attachment has the strongest attractive force of 7.4N and are recommended for use in 4-point or more implant supported overdentures.

The keeper screw for implants is tightened directly on the implant or screwed on top of an abutment ring. For example, for Brånemark compatible systems, the abutment ring is available in three different heights of 3.0mm, 4.0mm, and 5.5mm to compensate for the height of the gingiva.

Magnetic attachments for implants are compatible with major implant systems such as Brånemark, 3i, ITI and others. In terms of loosening prevention of the keeper screw, as shown in (Fig 4), sufficient drawback torque is designed into the mechanism. Also, as shown in (Fig 5), there is precise fit between the abutment and the implant fixture is only 1.7μm so that it may not become a place for the collection of bacteria.

In summary, the features of Magfit are

- Vastly improved attractive force through computer-aided optimization
- Perfect corrosion prevention through micro-laser welding technology and stainless steel casing
- Wide range of products available for different clinical applications.

Other Magnetic Attachment Systems

Other magnetic attachments currently available are Hitachi, Dyna, Steco and others.

These products are collectively shown in Table 2. All these products adopt laser welding to prevent the corrosion problem[7].

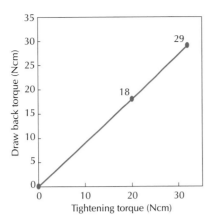

Fig 4 The relationship between tightening torque and draw-back torque.

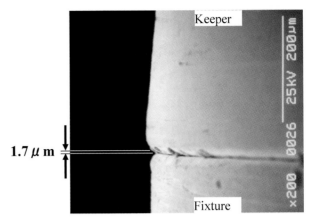

Fig 5 Gap between implant fixture and keeper.

Table 2: Other magnetic attachments.

Products	Magnetic assembly		Keeper		Height in total (mm)	Attractive force (N)	Attractive force performance (N/mm³)	Remarks
	Magnetic structure	Dimensions (mm)	Coping method	Dimensions (mm)				
Hyper Slim	Closed cap	ø 4.0 × 1.3	Cast Root Keeper Direct Bond	ø 4.0 × 0.8	2.1	6.5	0.25	Undercut
Dyna System	Opened cap	ø 4.0 × 1.5	Root Keeper Implant	ø 4.0 × 1.3	2.8	2.1	0.06	Flange Corrosive
Steco-Titanimagnetics	Opened cap	ø 4.8 × 2.6	Root Keeper Screw	ø 4.8 × 4.5	7.1	1.7	0.01	Undercut
Magna-Cap	Opened cap	ø 4.5 × 3.2	Cast Root Keeper Screw	ø 4.4 × 0.8	4.0	4.0	0.07	Flange
Micro Plant	Opened cap	ø 4.4 × 3.0	Screw	ø 4.2 × 5.0	8.0	1.5	0.01	Sandblasted

Hitachi

These magnetic attachments are developed for natural tooth roots. With a cap-type structure, the available attractive force range is 2.3N to 10.8N and the diameter range is 2.5mm to 5.5mm with a total of eight types. As shown in (Fig6), the attractive force is 20% less compared to Magfit of the same diameter.

Dyna

This magnetic attachment is mainly used for implant systems. Structurally, it is an open circuit design so the attractive force is inferior to a closed magnetic circuit. In order to prevent the corrosion problem, a stainless steel cap covers the magnet and is laser-welded on the side. But the laser welded parts shows lower quality which leads to a higher chance for corrosion. Market

evaluation shows that it is easy to corrode after prolonged use.

Steco

This magnetic attachment is mainly for implant applications. It is an open circuit type which needs to use 2 magnets. Compared to Magfit, the attractive force per volume is lower. However, it should be noted that an innovative improvement in terms of corrosion resistance is the casing made of titanium. There are flat, dome, or precision type magnets which has a rigidity function.

Magnacap, and others

These magnetic attachments are for natural tooth roots. In terms of price, they occupy a lower price range but they are susceptible to cor-

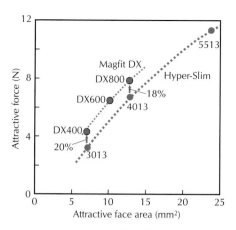

Fig6 Comparison of attractive force between Magfit DX and Hyper-Slim magnetic attachments.

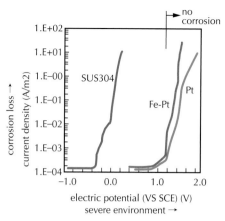

Fig7 Corrosion resistance of Fe-Pt.

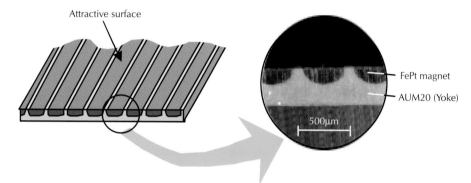

Fig8 Structure of FePt magnetic assembly.

rosion and low attractive force.

Promising Development of the Super Thin Magnetic Attachment

The Platinum-Iron (PtFe) magnet is a magnet alloy which has the potential attractive force equal to a NdFeB magnet. And moreover the PtFe magnet has the same corrosion characteristic as Pt metal (Fig7), and is a very safe alloy. Recently, by utilizing physical vapor deposition process, the PtFe magnet in the shape of a film which has an excellent maximum energy product of $159KJ/^3$ was invented. This value is about half the performance of a NdFeB. The development of a super-thin shape magnetism attachment is progressing very quickly[8]. The structure of this magnetic attachment is very unique, and as shown in (Fig8), it is the integrated structure of many minute magnets. With super-thin magnets, the attractive force per unit volume is about 10 times larger than the current Magfit which would

make it a great technological advancement in the field of magnetic attachments. Currently, the attractive force is about 3.8N. For reference, a super-thin shape magnetic attachment is shown in (Fig9) as compared with a Magfit. Furthermore, since it is thin, it can be bent easily.

The application of these super-thin type magnetic attachment is expected to make a denture retainer with use of vital teeth, beyond its current limitation of root cap attachments in which the crown part of the tooth needs to be cut off. Since the thickness of the magnetic structure and keeper is only 0.20mm and 0.05mm respectively, it can adhere with metal bond to the tooth after grinding the tooth enamel about 0.2mm. By combining Super-Thin magnetic attachments with conventional mechanical retainers such as clasps or conical telescope crowns, it can be possible to develop a simple, hybrid type functional retainer in which magnetic retention is used as a complementary function.

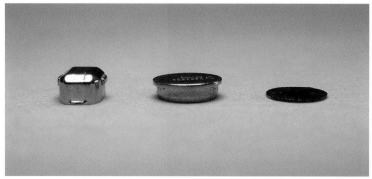

Fig 9 super-thin magnetic attachment compared with current products of Magfit EX and DX. assembly.

References

1. Tanaka Y, Nakamura Y, Desaki Y, Aizawa H, Ozawa T, Hiranuma K, Arai K, Fujii H, Honkura Y: Development of MAGFIT-EX SYSTEM as a Second Generation of the Magnetic Attachment. J J Mag Dent, 5(1): 24-30, 1996 (English abstract).

2. Toyoma H, Oyama T, Satoh Y, Oki K, Arai K: Develop and Clinical Application of Magnetic Attachment with Stress Breaker. pp. 80-85. In Ai,M. and Hiranuma,K. (eds.) Clinical Application of Magnetic Attachments. Japan, Quintessence, 2000.

3. Tanaka J: MRI Non-Interfering Magnetic Attachments. pp.96-103. In Ai M and Hiranuma K (eds.) Clinical Application of Magnetic Attachments. Japan, Quintessence, 2000.

4. Mizutani H: A Magnetic Attachment for Immediate Denture Repair in Aged Society. The Quintessence, 20(1), 199-205, 2001.

5. Arai K, Honkura Y: Development of Magnetic Attachment for Dental Implant, Intermag 2003, 1, 2003.

6. Maeda Y, Horisaka M, Matsuda S, Sogou M: The retainer of Implant Overdentures. J. Dental Tec., Extra issue 2004: 32-35, 2004.

7. Blankenstein Felix H.: Systemborstellungen. pp39-53. In Blankenstein, Felix H. (ed.) Magnete in der Zahnmedizin, flohr verlag. Germany, flohr verlag, Rottweil, 2001.

8. Aoyama H, Honkura Y: Magnetic Properties of Fe-Pt Sputtered Thick Film Magnet. J. Mag. in Jpn., 20(2): 237-240, 1996.

Part 2

Clinical Application of Magnetic Attachment

Chapter 7

A concept of designing dentures and role of the magnetic attachment

Minoru Ai

The magnetic attachment is a kind of root surface retentive appliances. The concept and requirement of designing dentures with magnetic attachments are not appreciably different from those of conventional removable partial dentures. But, since the attachment has unique properties in its retentive function caused by magnet, there may be a special requirement in its application. Before discussing design of the dentures with magnetic attachments, the author would like to briefly explain the basic problems in removable partial dentures.

The Aim of Prosthetic Treatment

Loss of the tooth is mostly caused by caries, periodontal disease, injuries and tumors. Current spread of oral hygiene knowledge has greatly controlled the occurrence of caries and periodontal disease, but tendency of the tooth loss is scarcely changed yet. Loss of only a tooth permits neighboring and opposing teeth to drift or extrude as time goes by and finally destroys occlusal relationship of whole teeth. These process may affect oral health and esthetic harmony and disturb oral functions of mastication and speech. When a number such as teeth are lost and not replaced, morphological and functional disturbances come to be more serious. The aim of prosthetic treatment is just to restore these damaged morphology and function by replacing lost tissues and to prevent the succeeding destructive process.

But, there is another aim. That is to maintain the restored condition for as long a period as possible as preventing damage to existing tissues. No matter how well the denture is functioning, if the abutments or soft tissue are damaged, the treatment can not be considered successful. Clinicians should pay particular attention to designing dentures to achieve both aims.

A Concept of Designing Dentures

In order to make such dentures as are fairly stable and function well for a long time, it is primarily important that the dentures should be designed based on the extensive knowledge of the clinical dentistry.

Removable partial dentures are supported by two different types of tissues, the remaining teeth, strictly the periodontal ligaments and the soft tissue of the residual alveolar ridge. They act quite differently in response to various mechanical and physical stimuli. The soft tissue displaces much more than the teeth on pressure. The amount of their displacement on pressure is significant. During mastication, dentures may move variously on the soft tissue as transmitting undesirable lateral force on the abutments. The undesirable force may bring about mobility of the abutments or worsen it, and furthermore may even destroy retentive appliances of the denture. Consequently, reduction of these movements of dentures is essential to protect the remaining tissues as well as prostheses (*Fig 1*).

Besides, the difference of the displacement

makes it difficult to keep a balance of occlusion between the remaining teeth and artificial teeth of the denture. The occlusal contacts loosen as the denture displaces on the soft tissue. There fore, it is necessary to consider the distribution of occlusal force to remaining teeth, especially abutments and underlying soft tissues in designing dentures.

In addition, morphological changes gradually take place in the denture supporting tissues even after insertion of the denture. They arise inevitably from aging process and pathological causes. According to this change, sinking and instability of the denture come out especially with tooth-tissue-supported dentures. The distal extension (free-end) denture, both Kennedy class 1 and 2, is a type of those dentures, which is supported with the abutment teeth at one end and with the residual ridge at the other. Sinking and instability of the denture worsen existing changes of the residual ridge in turn and bring about overload to the supporting teeth.

Fundamental Items for Designing Dentures

Removable partial dentures receive the force of various strength from different directions in oral functions. Vertical and horizontal forces attack to the denture from the opposing teeth, cheek or tongue even under the empty mouth condition, and the force of much bigger strength works on it through foods in mastication.

When making dentures, it should be considered that the denture has a resistible ability to these forces. That is three resisting functions such as "support", "retention" and "bracing" (*Fig2a–c*). Support is a function opposing to occlusal force to prevent the denture sinking, retention is a function against lifting force, and bracing is to prevent horizontal movements, rolling or dislodging of the dentures under occlusal force. In order to make the denture stable in function, it is essential that these functions

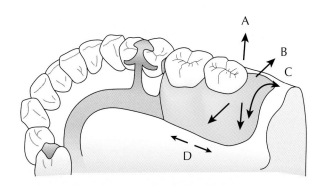

Fig 1 Four possible movements of a distal extension partial denture. A, Up-and-down movement. B, Lateral movement. C, Rotation around a longitudinal axis on the crest of the residual ridge. D, Antero-posterior movement or rotation around a vertical axis.

are assured in designing dentures.

a) Support

Concerning support of dentures, followings are to be considered.

- Imbalance or concentration of a load to the supporting tissues should be avoided. The soft tissue should be evenly pressed by the denture base in function.
- Occlusal force should be adequately distributed to the supporting tissues depending upon the bearing ability of each. Lateral force is unfavorable to the supporting tissues.
- The denture should be strongly constructed. If the denture bends easily by occlusal force, distribution of the force to the supporting tissues will be not done well as estimated.
- Connection of the denture to the abutment teeth should be determined with taking account of the amount of displacement of the soft tissue under the load and the size of denture bases. It is generally thought desirable that there is no play in the connection. Poor support could result in sinking of dentures and poor occlusal function.

b) Bracing

Bracing is borne mainly by the abutment teeth, but the stress caused by bracing could

Fig 2 Three actions required to a removable partial denture for its stability.

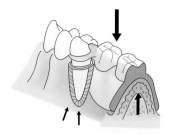

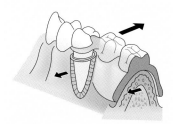

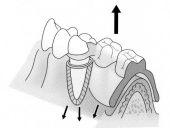

Fig 2a Support

Fig 2b Bracing

Fig 2c Retention

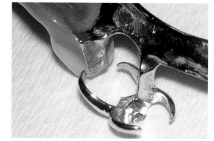

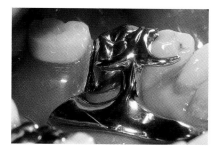

Fig 3a, b Minor connector and proximal plate working effectively for bracing.

a | b

Fig 3a Minor connector and proximal plate.
Fig 3b Minor connector and proximal plate fitted to the abutment.

bring about damage to the supporting tissues of the abutments. The followings are to be considered.

- Distribution of the occlusal force to the teeth and the denture-supporting soft tissue is important. Axial walls of the remaining teeth and slopes of the residual ridge are used for bracing.

- Each component part of dentures should be arranged so as to act effectively for bracing of dentures. Minor connectors and proximal plates work effectively for bracing (*Fig 3a, b*). Denture bases and major connectors fitted well to the soft tissues are also useful for bracing.

c) Retention

Retention of removable partial dentures is brought about mainly by the retentive appliances such as clasps, telescope crown and attachments. Remaining teeth, the residual ridge and the palate also contribute to retention of dentures with friction, mechanical interlocking and adhesion taking place between each component part of dentures and these oral tissues. The followings should be considered for retention of dentures.

- Retentive force of the denture should be distributed to each supporting tissue adequately. Retention relied on the retentive appliances alone is harmful to the abutment teeth. The denture should be retained as a whole by all the component parts of dentures.

- Load to the abutment teeth should be controlled, especially lateral force to the teeth should be managed as little as possible.

- Relationship between the denture bases and the underlying soft tissue is very important for retention of the denture. When the denture base fit well, it will sticks fast to the soft tissue and good retention can be obtained.

Fundamental Concept of Designing Dentures

In designing removable partial dentures, it is required that the denture is stable with its artificial teeth making a full dental arch together with remaining teeth and it keeps good function for a long time. In order to fulfill these requirements, it is essential that support, bracing and retention of the denture should work adequately as they are expected. But, oral conditions such as number and location of remaining teeth, morphology of the residual ridge, displacement of the soft tissue

Fig 4a, b Typical fixed bridge(a) and clasp-retained removable partial denture(b).

a | b

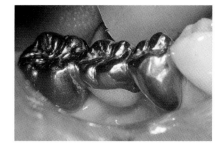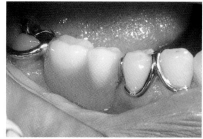

a | b

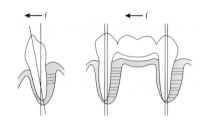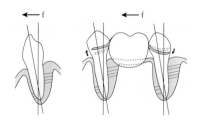

Fig 5a, b Possible behaviors of abutments of fixed bridge and removable partial denture under the lateral load(f). a. Fixed bridge. Abutments rotate laterally around apical axis but transfer sagittally. b. Removable partial denture. Abutments rotate apical axis in both directions.

under a load and occlusal relationship are greatly concerned with it.

a) Oral condition and stability of dentures

From the investigation with the life of prosthesis, the followings are indicated[1]. When not a few teeth remained, fixed or removable bridges, attachment retained dentures and strong-built metal frame dentures, which were rigidly connected by the abutment teeth, are generally long lived, while loosely connected dentures, like the denture with wrought-wire clasps, are short lived. In the case of few remaining teeth, however, the dentures borne by the soft tissue provided fairly good result.

b) Connection of dentures to the abutments

It is often experienced that fixed prosthesis is generally more successful than removable prosthesis. This mainly comes from the difference in the way of connection between prostheses and abutments. Fixed bridges are making one unit with the abutment teeth by solid retainers such as crowns (*Fig 4a, b*). When a bridge receives a load, the abutment teeth are forced to move together with the bridge itself (*Fig 5a, b*). In the case of a removable partial denture, the connection to the

abutment is loose, and the clasps slide on the axial surface of the abutment teeth with the movement of dentures and rock the teeth. Comparing with both cases, the amount of the periodontal ligaments working for the resistance is different. Supposing that same amount of a load is exerted, the stress of each ligament must be great with the abutment teeth of dentures compared with that of bridges. The abutment teeth of dentures will fall into the pathological conditions in a long time.

From this viewpoint, it is recommended that after the stability of denture bases ensured, the denture should be rigidly connected to the abutment teeth. This leads to the concept of "rigid-support".

"Rigid-support" means to support occlusion rigidly by using removable prosthesis. This concept is very important in keeping masticatory system in good condition.

The denture retained by telescope crowns is thought to be a typical rigid-support prosthesis[2]. They produce the similar effect as the fixed bridge and keep a long life[3].

The rigid-support is based on the condition that the mobility of denture base on the soft tissue is minimized. Therefore, this can be easily achieved in the tooth-supported denture, where

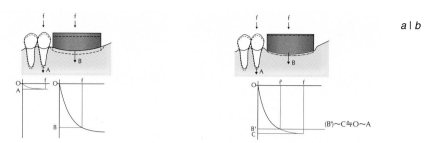

Fig 6a, b Adjustment of displacement of the teeth and the soft tissue under a load. a. Displacement of teeth and the denture base constructed on the model by static impression technique. When a force(f) works, the denture base sinks considerably(B) compared with teeth(A). b. Displacement of teeth and the denture base constructed on the model by pressure impression technique with a load(f'). The surface of the model is to be displaced to B'. When a force (f) works, the denture base sinks in nearly the same degree(C) as the teeth(A).

the soft tissue hardly participates in the support. But, how is it in the case of dentures partly or mainly supported by the soft tissue? If the denture mobility can be will controlled to the tolerance of periodontal ligaments, the same situation as in the tooth-supported denture will be theoretically established, and the rigid-support is to be achieved. The possibility of realization of this depends upon the dynamic property of the underlying soft tissue and how to deal with the tissue in making dentures.

Actually, this is realized by means that the denture base is determined as large as possible within the denture-supporting area, and the soft tissue is pressed in almost the same degree as in occlusal function and it is transfered to the working cast for making the denture (*Fig6a, b*). In order to obtain such the pressed soft tissue, the pressure impression technique, the modified altered cast technique are available.

However, there are a few cases with great displacement of the soft tissue under a load. In such cases, the rigid-support is not adaptable. Stress-breaking retainer may be necessary.

c) Retainers of overdentures

In the case of very few remaining teeth, over-denture is recommended, where telescope crowns or root surface attachments are in general applied as retainers (*Fig7a, b*). As mentioned above, telescope crowns are connected rigidly to the abutment to realize the rigid-support successfully.

Root surface attachments produce flexible connection. But, it rocks the abutment teeth less than other retainers in occlusal function, and the prognosis of the denture is almost favorable. Its main reason seems that the action point of the load is low on the cast base. In the case of magnetic attachments, rocking of the abutment teeth is much less, because the magnetic assembly easily slides on the keeper or separates from it, when the denture moves excessively.

In addition, the magnetic attachment is quite different from other retainers in its mechanism of retention. Its maximum retentive force is exerted, when the magnetic assembly keeps fast in contact with the keeper (*Fig8*). This means that in using the magnetic attachment as a retainer, it is essential for the denture to be as stable as possible. If a denture is unstable, the magnetic assembly always slides on the keeper. The retention of the denture will be reduced and the attractive surface of the attachment will be worn down as the result (*Fig9*). The magnetic attachment retained denture is not a rigid-support prosthesis but should be constructed according to the concept of rigid-support.

In any dentures borne by the soft tissue even partly, adequate impression technique and large denture base are essential to reduce the displacement of the dentures and to make application of rigid-support possible. These are thought to be a key to success in making the dentures.

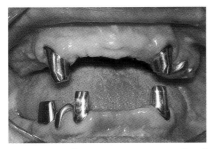
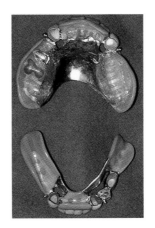
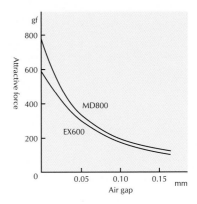

Fig 7a, b Telescope crown-retained overdentures. a. Inner crowns in the mouth. b. Inner surface of the upper and lower dentures.

Fig 8 Influence of air gap on the attractive force of magnetic attachments.

d) Occlusion of removable partial dentures

In order to minimize the denture mobility it is necessary to reduce especially the lateral component of the force as much as possible.

First of all, flat artificial posterior teeth are selected and arranged along on the ridge. In the intercuspal position, an even occlusal contact of the arch should be produced by artificial teeth together with remaining teeth, and the occlusal contact points of the artificial teeth should be adjusted so as to come over the ridge. Narrow occlusal surfaces are useful to reduce especially sinking of dentures. In the lateral or anterior jaw gliding, which frequently occur during mastication, artificial molars should not make occlusal contact, that is, disclusion of the posteriors is favorable. If canines or anterior teeth remain and work as a guidance of the jaw movement, the denture should be discluded. In short, the essencial point is to prevent the denture from the lateral as much as possible.

Requirements for Designing Dentures

The following conditions should be satisfied in designing dentures.

1. Minimizing denture mobility
2. Precautions against caries and periodontal disease
3. Countermeasure for break of dentures
4. Following the biological changes

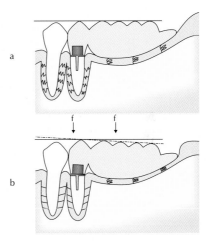

Fig 9 Effect of magnetic attachments and stability of dentures. a. The denture in a rest. b. The denture dislodged due to its unstable denture base under occlusal load. Magnetic attachment reduces its effect.

Minimizing Denture Mobility

Dentures should be designed so as to be as stable as possible during oral functions. Each component part of removable partial dentures works for support, bracing and retention of the dentures independently or in their combinations.

①Rest ·························· Support, (Bracing)

②Denture base ············

·········· Support, (Bracing, Retention)

③Minor connector, Proximal plate

······················ Bracing, (Retention)

④Major connctor ·········

·········· Support, (Bracing, Retention)

⑤Retainer ················ Retention, (Bracing)

Denture should be designed according to this

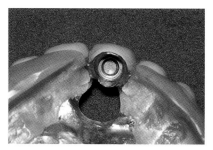 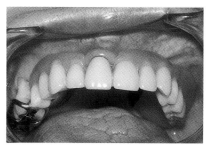 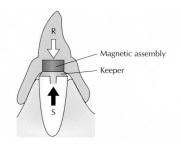

Fig 10a, b Opened marginal gingiva of the abutment of magnetic attachment. a. Inner surface of the denture. Gingiva adjacent to the abutment(right central incisor) is opened. b. The denture in the mouth. (Courtesy of Ishihata N, D.D.Sc.)   *a | b*

Fig 11 The denture with magnetic attachment is supported by the abutment root (S) and retained by the function of magnetic attachment (R).

order.

In order to reduce the denture mobility, following two points are required. One is to control the direction of the mobility and the other is to reduce the amount of the mobility. On the basis of these requirements, location of the abutment, area of the denture base, location and size of the minor connector and proximal plate should be determined. Retention of the denture should not be depended upon the retainers alone, because the abutment teeth are overloaded and their prognosis becomes very poor. It is desirable that even if retainers are lacked, the denture is kept up well with other component parts.

Precautions Against Caries and Periodontal Disease

It is often pointed out with denture wearers, that debris tends to accumulate at the remaining teeth and its neighboring soft tissue and caries and periodontal disease are aggravated as the result. In order to solve these problems, the following should be considered in designing dentures.

(1) Dentures are made in simple structure for ease to clean. Self-cleansing factor or materials easily kept clean should be taken into consideration.

(2) Marginal gingiva is opened, if possible. Because marginal gingiva is sensible for mechanical and biological stimuli and is liable to fall into inflammatory changes. In the case of overdenture, marginal gingiva is generally covered, but it is recommended to open this area, even partly

(*Fig 10a, b*).

The keeper of the magnetic attachment is fixed to the root surface through cast base or directly to the root with adhesive agents. Imperfect fit of the cast base or wrong cementing agent may cause secondary caries on the root surface. Adhesive resin cement is useful, especially such a resin cement as connects organically to the tooth substance has a great effect of caries prevention. In the Root Keeper system, this type of resin cement is essential.

Countermeasure for Break of Dentures

It is important that the denture is not easily broken or worn down in its use. The followings are especially emphasized for prevention of these discomforts.

(1) Concentration of the stress is to be avoided.

(2) Strong combination of materials is needed.

With magnetic attachment applications, shedding of the magnetic assembly from the denture is the most of the troubles. This is caused by concentration of the stress at the point of the attachment on the denture base, poor adhesion technique as well as faulty physical properties of the adhesive agents.

Following the Biological Changes

Denture supporting tissues gradually change even after insertion of the denture.

The denture should be designed in the structure beforehand so as to be easily adjusted or

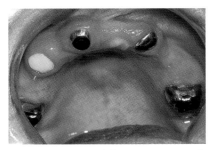 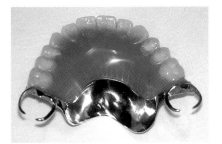 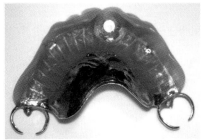

Fig 12a–c A case of the magnetic attachment used together with clasps. a. The magnetic attachment applied for the right central incisor. b. The denture with two clasps and magnetic attachment. c. Inner surface of the denture.

a | b | c

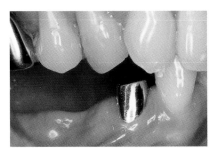 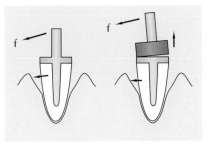 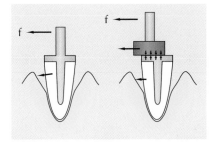

Fig 13 An abutment of magnetic attachment. The root surface is prepared above the level of gingiva for bracing. (Courtesy of Mizutani H, D.D.Sc.)

Fig 14a, b Function of magnetic attachments to a leaning force(a) and a lateral force(b). When the force is exerted, other retainers transfer it directly to the abutment(left a,b), while magnetic attachments scarcely transfer it due to its dislocation(right a) or slide(right b).

a | b

repaired as following the biological changes.

Application of Magnetic Attachment and its Effect

The concept and requirements for designing dentures have been explained. They can be applied to the dentures with magnetic attachments as they are.

The "Magnetic Attachment" Retainer

The magnetic attachment is a type of retentive appliance of dentures. It is unique in its function. Retentive appliances generally have combined function of support, bracing and retention. The magnetic attachment also has these functions as the root surface attachment, but it is different in functions of bracing and retention from other retainers. Firm support is expected because the magnetic attachment transmits occlusal force to the root (*Fig 11*). But, it does not have distinct bracing ability due to the nature of magnet. Retention is adequately obtained because the retentive force of magnetic attachments is determined distinctly. At present, the retentive force of

4–10N is reported.

a) Retentive force

The retentive force of magnetic attachments is brought about by attraction of the magnet. It decreases rapidly with the gap between attractive surfaces of the magnetic assembly and the keeper. For instance, gap of 0.1mm makes the retentive force reduce to a half of the maximum, as shown in *Fig 8*. Accordingly, great care is necessary for setting the magnetic attachment. The retentive force works widely, but the force being parallel to the attractive surface is 1/6-1/10 of the vertical force. This is the reason of weak bracing ability of magnetic attachments.

The retentive force of wide range is very useful as the retainer of the dentures. It can be used almost free from the path of insertion of the dentures. Consequently, the magnetic attachment can be easily used together with other retainers, and this is one of its advantages (*Fig 12a–c*).

b) Bracing of dentures with magnetic attachments

Fig 15 The tooth with big C-R ratio used for the abutment of magnetic attachment. The tooth is cut at the level of the marginal gingiva after root treatment.

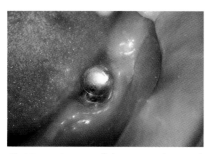 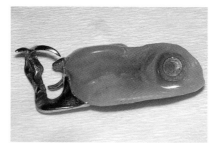 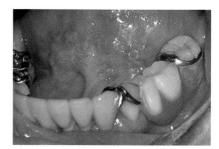

Fig 16a~c A case of the magnetic attachment used for the last molar. a. The abutment of the last molar. b. Inner surface of the repaired denture. c. The denture in the mouth.

a | b | c

When the magnetic attachment is applied to removable partial dentures or overdentures, since the bracing function is scarcely expected with magnetic attachments, it must be provided with other component parts of the denture. The bracing effect is usually secured by the denture base or the connectors. If the abutment tooth can bear the lateral force, the bracing effect is incorporated by preparing the root surface above the level of the gingiva and reinforced (*Fig 13*).

c) Protection of abutment teeth

The weak bracing effect is certainly disadvantage as the retainer for making denture stability. But, this is great advantage in respect of protection of the abutments from destructive lateral forces (*Fig 14a, b*). This can not be obtained with other retainers. Because of this protective property, the teeth with unfavorable periodontal conditions or short roots, or even fractured teeth are allowed to be used as abutments. With these abutments, the root surface should be usually prepared as low as possible in order to minimize lateral loads on the roots.

In addition, it is significant for preservation of their supporting tissues that abutment teeth are kept for a long time by reduction of the lateral stress. Especially, preservation of the periodontal ligaments including sensory nerves is valuable for control of occlusal force and maintenance of harmonious masticatory function.

When the denture is moving considerably, clasps or telescope crowns work actively with their strong retentive functions. They are apt to bring undesirable stress on the abutments. On the other hand, magnetic attachments reduce their function as the contact between the attractive surfaces is broken. As for the function of retainers, the magnetic attachment can be said as protective type of retentive appliance.

d) Advantages and disadvantages

Advantages and disadvantages of the magnetic attachment and its application are summarized as follows.

Advantages:

① Precise retentive force is obtained. The retention is constant and permanent.

② It protects the abutment teeth. It can be used for even the teeth with negative factors for other retainers.

③ The path of insertion is not precise. It can be easily used together with other retainers.

④ It is suitable for the aged and the handicapped

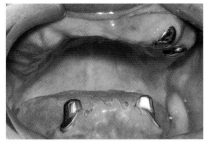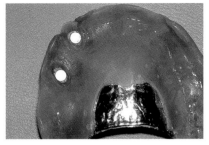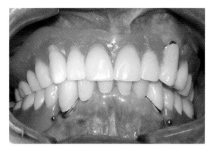

Fig 17a–c A case of the magnetic attachment used in the upper overdenture. a. Left canine and the second premolar used for the abutments. b. Inner surface of the overdenture. c. The denture in the mouth.

a | b | c

Fig 18a, b A case of the magnetic attachment used together with clasps as a indirect retainer. a. Inner surface of the distal extension denture. Magnetic attachment is used on the first premolar. b. Indirect retainer applied for the teeth on the other side. (Courtesy of Mizutani H, D.D.Sc.)

a | b

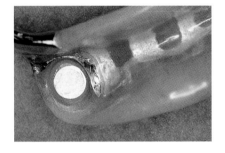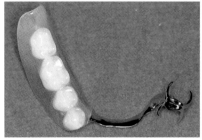

patients, because the denture insertion and removal is easy for the patients.

⑤ It can be instantly used as a substitute retainer in the repair of being used denture.

Disadvantages:

① It can not be used for intact teeth with sound crowns.

② Its bracing function is very little.

③ The technique looks so simple that it is liable to be used carelessly.

Application of the Magnetic Attachment

The magnetic attachment has many advantages as retentive appliances, but the application is somewhat limited because of the need of devitalization and decoronation of the abutment teeth.

a) Indication for the abutment teeth

Magnetic attachments can be applied on the cases to which the conventional retainers can not be used, such as teeth with advanced bone resorption, mobility or short roots. Its application is also beneficial in the case of a few remaining teeth with mobility or too big crown-root ratio[4, 5] (*Fig 15*). Prognosis of the teeth with only horizontal mobility is favorable.

b) Application for removable partial dentures

Magnetic attachments are often used together with clasps or telescope crowns for removable partial dentures, and there are two cases in its use. One is the use for repairing dentures (*Fig 16a–c*). The dentures can be easily modified with using magnetic attachments, when some repairs are required due to failure of existing retainers or destruction of the abutment teeth. Replacing the existing retainer with a magnetic attachment is quite easy because it is less sensitive to the path of insertion. This enables the magnetic attachment to be used together with other retentive appliances. Almost one half of the magnetic attachment applications today are said to be in this category. As the existing denture already settles well, application of the attachment is easy.

Another case is the use of magnetic attachments for new dentures. When the roots of the teeth which have been used as the abutment of crown or bridge remain among a few remaining teeth, magnetic attachments can be applied together with other retainers. The denture should be made according to the concept and the requirements previously mentioned. The new dentures mainly supported by the soft tissue are apt to sink with the displacement of the tissue under occlusal load. Therefore, it is extremely important to deal with the differential displacement between the remaining roots and the soft tissue precisely for reduction of the sinking of dentures and for protection of the abutment roots from overstress. Furthermore, the magnetic assembly should be fixed after the denture settles down sufficiently in the mouth. If the magnetic assembly is fixed in the laboratory process, the following troubles may come out after insertion of dentures. That is, owing to the sinking of the denture base, the abutment roots are strongly pressed with pain, the retention of the denture decreases due to separation of the magnetic assembly from the keeper, or severe wears occur partly on the attractive surfaces of the attachment. In order to avoid these troubles, it is recomended to fix the magnetic assembly at chairside after trying the denture without it for 1 or 2 weeks.

c) Application for the overdentures

The magnetic attachment is often applied to overdentures as well. When a removable partial denture is converted to a overdenture using magnetic attachments, satisfactory results are obtained in most cases (*Fig 17a–c*). The remaining teeth are preserved by root treatment and used as the abutments for the magnetic attachments. This can be said as the most suitable way of application for magnetic attachments. In designing the magnetic attachiment retained overdenture, care should be taken of the support of dentures, which is the same as the case of new removable partial dentures. The support must be distributed to both of the abutments and the soft tissue.

The overdenture with magnetic attachments is not a rigid-support denture because it is not united with the abutment teeth into one unit. However, the concept of rigid-support should be applied in making the denture. When the denture moves excessively, the attachment loses its function by breaking off the contact of the attractive surfaces and the denture is dislodged. Therefore, the denture must be made as stable as possible in function. Impression technique and fixing process of the magnetic assembly are very important.

Arrangement of the Magnetic Attachments and the Denture Stability

For the retention and the stability of dentures, number and arrangement of the abutments are important rather than the amount of retentive force of the retainers fixed to them. As mentioned previously, it is desirable for the protection of the abutment teeth that the retentive force of the retainer is in enough degree for making up for the lack of the retention of the denture by other component parts. If a certain amount of occlusal force is exerted, the more the number of abutments is, the less the load on each abutment becomes. However, the number should be reduced to the minimum to simplify the denture structure.

For the abutment of the magnetic attachment, canines are used most often. The reason is that they remain long with their steady roots. They are not selected according to the design of dentures.

It is so advantageous that the area surrounded by the line which connects the abutment teeth is large for the stability and retention of the dentures. Although this is the fundamental principle of the design of conventional partial dentures, it is not realistic for the magnetic attachment dentures where the abutment teeth are applied only to the residual roots. But it can attain by using indirect retainers such as clasps together when some teeth remain (*Fig 18a, b*)

Summary

In this chapter, the concept and requirements

necessary for designing dentures with magnetic attachments have been explained. The magnetic attachment is a retentive appliance unique in its function and has many advantages. The denture should be made on the basis of these concepts and requirements and the magnetic attachment should be applied so as to make good use of its advantages. If they are put into practice properly, the denture with the magnetic attchment will be accepted by patients with great satisfaction.

References

1. McGivney G P, Carr A B : McCracke's Removable Partial Prosthodontics. 10th ed. Mosby, St Louis, 2000.
2. Körber E : Die prothetische Versorgung des Lückenge-bisses. Behunderhebung und Planung. 3 Auflage, München Wien, Carl Hanser Verlag, 1987.
3. Körber K H : Konuskronen-Das rationelle Teleskopsystem. Einführung in Klinik und Technik. 5 Auflage, Heidelberg, A.Hüthig Verlag, 1983.
4. Ishihata N, Mizutani H, Ai M : Application of ferro-magnetic alloy for prosthodontics, Part 5. Application of magnetic attachment for prosthodontically hopeless teeth. J Jpn Prosthodont Soc, 31: 1445−1453, 1987 (English abstract).
5. Ishihata N, Mizutani H, Nakamura K, Ishikawa S, Suzuki Y, Ai M : Clinical application making the best use of the properties of the dental magnet. J J Mag Dent, 1: 88−98, 1992 (English abstract).

Chapter 8

Preparations of abutments for magnetically retained overdentures

Hiroshi Mizutani / Vygandas Rutkunas

Introduction

One of the most responsible steps in overdenture fabrication is preparation of abutment teeth. In most situations the operator will have little choice, as there is seldom an abundance of abutment candidates. Inadequate abutment preparation may complicate following clinical and laboratory steps, threat the prognosis of abutments, influence the overdenture performance and diminish insertion period. Since abutments supporting overdenture are commonly the only few left teeth, they usually have compromised periodontal and endodontic conditions, and are affected by caries and undergone extensive restorative procedures. Necessarily vital questions arise - to use remaining teeth as a support for overdenture or to extract them and if it is decided to fabricate teeth supported overdenture - how to select abutments. Judging suitability of abutments periodontal and supporting bone status, mobility, endodontic aspects, root morphology and location of them have to be evaluated.

Periodontal Considerations and Support

Abutments showing vertical mobility are subjected to extractions. The statement that remaining teeth limit resorption of residual ridges is valid when there are no signs of periodontal pathology. On the contrary keeping the teeth with periodontitis can enhance resorption of ridges. Thus the periodontal condition of abut-

ments is a critical region and future success or failure of restoration can be judged roughly from state of it. Diminishing the coronal height of the abutment tooth favors in lowering stress on abutment and improving periodontal condition. The supporting bone height have to be evaluated using radiographs, also as it is considered complete mouth rehabilitation the panoramic radiographs are preferable. Unfortunately as prognosis of abutments depends on many factors there are no forthright guidelines suggesting height of abutment preparation according to the available bone support. The single rooted teeth are more suitable candidates. Due to more favorable bone architecture of mandibular bone than of maxillary the mandibular teeth retained overdenture is considered to be more predictable and requiring less number of abutments treatment option. However if there are no choice multi-rooted teeth even with furcations involved using root separation and/or resection and appropriate abutment preparation can be suitable for overdenture retention. Overdenture abutments demand scrupulous hygiene and if inter-dental space between two abutment teeth is too small special measures have to be taken to ensure proper hygiene or to extract more unfavorable one. A maxillary bone have less density thus provides lesser amount of support. It is recommended to use more than 2 abutments retaining maxillary overdenture. Nevertheless it is very difficult to evaluate apart the stability of abutments gained due to favorably changed crown-root ratio and beneficial influence of attachment type. Usually the available teeth for overdenture retention are canines. But utilizing extra abutments can have advantage of increased stability and lower load on abutments as it enables more rigid design of overdenture. Utilizing magnetic attachments the unique opportunity of "bracing without retention" can be employed thus stress on abutments is controlled more easily. The ideal number of attachments for a lower overdenture according to Brewer and Morrow is four and they should be evenly distributed in the arch, e.g. two canines and two molars (preferable second molars) for maximum support. Though rigid designs are slightly more preferred by patients but the superiority of them is not significant. In case natural teeth fail to qualify as abutments for overdenture support the implant option can be weighted. Implant retained overdentures have been approved as highly successful and predictable treatment method. Yet proprioception, which is not available with implants, plays very important role in controlling masticatory movements and patients with implants can face more difficult initial period for adaptation. Also proprioception of natural teeth act like a cutout for excessive stresses on abutments. Magnetic attachments owing their ability to break lateral force easily and preserve periodontaly weakened teeth are more often prescribed for abutments with mobility and enable the overdenture treatment option while other types of attachments can not be utilized in these cases. Similarly it could be used with implants of length which can be considered as too short for retain overdenture by mechanical attachments. There is suggested opinion that implant supported mandibular overdentures may improve masticatory performance only in persons with a less than adequate mandibular ridge, while with sufficient height of mandibular ridge (2.1-2.8 mm) the difference is not significant.

Endodontic Considerations

As root cap design for magnetic attachments have low profile the abutment teeth have to be treated endodontically. Endodontic treatment in overdenture patient could be quite complicated as the abundance of secondary dentine and consequent narrowing of root canal is commonly observed phenomenon. It should be avoided of leaving vital teeth as abutments even if the recession of pulp cavity is advanced and/or root canals are very narrow because the secondary dentin does not form perfect seal. If it was failed to complete endodontic treatment the additional sealing agents and periodic radiological examination should be employed. Also adequate temporary and permanent sealing of canal is required.

Hygiene

Overdenture treatment modality is quite specific due to covering of abutment teeth with denture base thus interrupting saliva flow and other self-cleaning mechanisms of oral cavity. Also temperature and micro-flora changes are the risk factors for periodontal health. All mentioned above factors claim higher requirements for overdenture abutment coping restoration rather than for any other type of it. The selection and preparation of abutment teeth should allow proper oral hygiene and placed restoration should not jeopardize it. As it was mentioned above the proper distance between abutments is required in order to use inter-dental brush etc.

Vertical Space

Another important factor that should be considered is vertical space available. Even with periodontaly sound teeth the high abutment restorations providing bracing as well as support are not feasible if the vertical space is not suffice. Owing to extremely small vertical dimension magnetic attachments are easily applicable in majority of these cases. The magnetic attachment could be

Fig 1a−c Preparations for with-leg keeper (44).

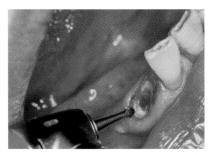

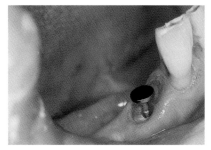

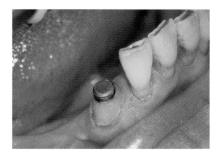

Fig 1a Carious tissue was perfectly removed by round bur.

Fig 1b Try-in root keeper into prepared root tooth. The surface of the keeper should be parallel to the occlusal plane and be positioned in appropriate level to provide inter-occlusal space needed.

Fig 1c Root keeper with dual cure resin cap set in the mouth.

shorter than any other stud-attachments in the world, because it has no process or dimple. However, it could be still a problem since the considerable space needed is for denture base and artificial teeth to cover the root cap sometimes. Cup type design of magnetic attachments allow smaller vertical space (but occupy larger occlusal area) and can be more handy when vertical space is restricted. Using thin metal denture base can solve the problem also. The minimum vertical space required is approximately 3 mm in anterior and 4 mm in posterior regions.

Abutment Tooth Preparation

Despite abutment preparations for root caps could look quite similar to ones for ordinary post-and-cores or root caps for mechanical attachments at the first glance, however it involves some specific aspects.

The versatile use of magnetic attachments dictates different preparation techniques depending on the way they are used. In all of the cases it has to be assumed that magnetic attachments posses minimal thickness and maximally preserve hard tissues. Keeper is a part of magnetic attachment, which is attached to the abutment. There are several ways to attach keeper to the abutment tooth and preparation will depend upon:

- With root keeper system.
- Cast-bonded keeper system.

- Tray-in keeper system.

First of all, carious tissues and remaining restorations have to be carefully removed. If a sound tooth crown is remaining it should be removed too, unless endodontic treatment is not planed. Remaining crown is useful during endodontic treatment as it aids as orientation for root canal direction. If the bracing is not desired the level of 1 mm above gingival margin is preferred.

With Root Keeper System *(Fig 1a−c)*

It was one of the first techniques offered for attaching keeper to the abutment. Keeper with attached prefabricated post is cemented to the root (core built-up is accomplished at the same time). The magnetic attachments exhibit best retentive properties when they are oriented parallel to occlusal surface and more than 10° inclination is considered to have adverse effect on retentive properties of magnetic attachment. Thus post attached to the keeper is made flexible in order to orientate surface of the keeper as parallel to occlusal surface as possible. The preparation technique is quite straightforward and mainly is governed by carious tissues removal and gaining appropriate vertical high. The use of special designed burs corresponding in size with keeper and post is recommended. However this method does not have good long-term results - the sur-

Fig 2a–c Preparations for cast-bonded keeper (47).

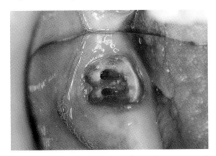

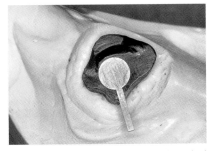

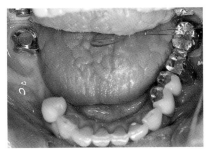

Fig 2a Carious removed and prepared root tooth for cast-bonded keeper.

Fig 2b Wax pattern with cast bonded keeper. The keeper is placed below the level of distal gingival margin to obtain enough inter-occlusal space, besides minimum 0.3 mm thickness of wax between keeper and tooth structures is required for proper casting.

Fig 2c Root cap with keeper and magnetic assembly in the mouth. The magnetic surface set on the keeper is the same level to the distal gingival margin.

Fig 3a–c Preparations for tray-in keeper (14).

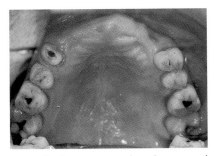

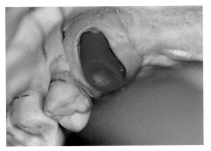

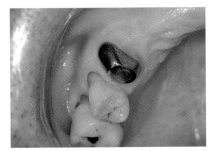

Fig 3a Carious removed and prepared root tooth for tray-in keeper. Preparation is entirely the same as the ordinary one since the keeper is not involved in the wax pattern.

Fig 3b Wax pattern with tray-in keeper. The occlusal level of the tray and wax should be the same.

Fig 3c Root cap with cement-bonded keeper set in the mouth.

face roughness of build-up material is associated with accumulation of denture plaque, also it can be cracked, worn or de-solved and secondary caries can appear. Depending on the amount of remaining dentin and vertical space available there could be distinguished two modifications: cement -in and cement-on. In the first the recess for placing keeper on the surface of abutment root is created and in the second - keeper with post is cemented without preparing recess in the root, just on the top of it.

Cast-bonded Keeper System *(Fig 2a–c)*

Since this cast-bonded technique involve fabrication of metal root coping (root cap) the preparation involves placing chamfered margin in the level of marginal gingiva and creating slightly divergent walls of root canal and slightly convergent for the axial walls (around 15°). Due to low lateral forces transferred to abutments the dowel post can be shorter - about 5mm and less. Also ferrule effect is useful in protection of abutments when caries extends to subgingival margin its not feasible to place it. Anti-rotational notch is made usually on the lingual side of root canal. Root cap embeds keeper, which should be surrounded by proper thickness of metal, otherwise the possibility of casting defects will be high. It is recommended to keep minimum wax thickness of 0.3 mm around keeper thus corresponding reduction of inner surface of the abutment root have to be accomplished especially in cases of restricted vertical dimension. Also special alloys as Fe-Pt can be used for custom made keeper, yet due to lower ferromagnetic properties of alloys their use is limited. The internal root surface should correspond to form of keeper as it enables lower placement of it and gaining vertical space as well. Then preparation is finished with fine diamonds and the sharp angles are smoothened.

Tray-in Keeper System *(Fig3a–c)*

According to this tray-in keeper system, metal root cap has no keeper immediately after cast, and finished metal cap is entirely the same as the ordinary one except cementing the keeper. Thus, preparation of tray-in keeper is also the same as the ordinary one and is referred to the cast-bonded keeper system.

References

1. Preiskel H W : Overdentures Made Easy. A Guide to Implant and Root Supported Prostheses. London, Quitessence Books, 1996.
2. Hou G L, Tsai C C, Weisgold A S : Treatment of molar furcation involvement using root separation and a crown and sleeve-coping telescopic denture. A longitudinal study. J Periodontol. Sep, 70(9): 1098–1109, 1999.
3. Mizutani H : Consideration of support, bracing, retention of removable partial denture. pp201–210. In Mizutani H and Hoshino E (eds.) Evaluation of Removable Partial Dentures. Tokyo, The Nippon Dental Review, 1995.
4. Brewer A A, Morrow R M : Overdentures (2nd ed.). St. Louis, Toronto, London, Mosby, 1980.
5. Dudic A, Mericske-Stern R : Retention mechanisms and prosthetic complications of implant-supported mandibular overdentures: long-term results. Clin Implant Dent Relat Res, 4(4): 212–219, 2002.
6. Kimoto K, Garrett N R : Effect of mandibular ridge height on masticatory performance with mandibular conventional and implant-assisted overdentures. Int J Oral Maxillofac Implants, Jul-Aug, 18(4): 523–530, 2003.
7. Dias A P, Honkura Y : Retentive prostheses with magnets. Proceedings of the Symposium on Magnetic Attachment System Organized by Hong Kong Prosthetic Dentistry Society, May, 1998.
8. Mizutani H, Nishiyama A, Yatabe M, et al: Influence of directional variations of keeper on magnetic attractive force. J Dent Res, 82 (special Issue): C-399, 2003.

Chapter 9

Cast base (Coping) system

Hiroshi Mizutani / Vygandas Rutkunas

Introduction

Root cap containing keeper can be fabricated using two different techniques: cast-bonded and cement-bonded keeper techniques. In the first way, keeper is attached to the root cap mechanically. Keeper is added to the wax pattern of the root cap prior to casting and after casting the keeper remains in the root cap. Keeper material has to have higher melting temperature than dental alloy of the root cap going to be cast from. During crystallization root cap undergoes shrinkage which is smaller than that of prefabricated keeper (SUS 447J1 or SUS444 alloys) as it was not melted. As a result keeper remains firmly pressed in the root cap (*Fig 1*).

Another option is to attach keeper to the root cap after casting by cement. The cast root cap is finished and polished and keeper cemented into specially prepared recess in the top of the root cap. The method is called cement-bonded or heatless keeper technique (*Fig 2*).

Special alloys possessing soft ferromagnetic properties were also proposed for root cap casting. In this case root cap itself has all features required for the keeper. Retentive force provided by magnetic attachments depends on the size of the keeper, thus root cap cast with ferromagnetic alloy should enhance retentive force considerably. Ferritic or martensitic stainless steel, Pd-Co-Pt, Permendur, Cr-Mo and other ferromagnetic alloys had been used for casting root caps. The Fe-Pt alloy with 69% of Fe produces high magnetic saturation values and great attractive force; they have a potential to serve as magnetic attachment keepers. Higher amount of Fe determines advantageous ferromagnetic properties but decreases anticorrosion resistance, while Pt increases anticorrosive properties and favors on casting. However the ferromagnetic properties of these alloys are inferior to those of prefabricated keeper and results in lower retentive force. Besides, the melting temperature of those alloys is very high (over 1,200°C) and that make it difficult to cast and/or achieve marginal fit. Therefore ferromagnetic alloys for keeper casting are not used widely.

Laboratory Procedure

Prefabricated keepers made from stainless steel (SUS 447J1or SUS444) are widely used[1] because of simple laboratory technique. However, due to sensitivity to high temperatures and difference in electrochemical potentials of casting alloys and keeper materials, proper laboratory protocol should be followed in order to obtain high-grade cast-keeper interface. The improper casting, pickling with acids and/or polishing can result in diminished attractive force and corrosion resistance.

Dental Alloys

There are no special requirements for root cap casting alloys. Keeper materials are not sensitive to high temperatures as permanent magnets;

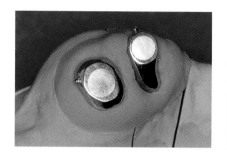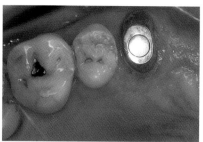

Fig 1 Working model with silicone gum. Root caps with cast-bonded keepers.
Fig 2 Root cap with cement-bonded keeper in situ.

1 | 2

however the overheating of keeper should be avoided. Overheating of keeper may cause oxidization and diminish resistance to corrosion as well[2]. Also casting alloy should be precise enough as root cap has thin sections, which is difficult to cast. Casting has to result in intimate contact of metal alloy and keeper. Presence of crevice between them will be the reason of crevice corrosion and colour changes. Type IV gold alloy and 12% gold-silver-palladium alloy highly recommended for root cap casting. They have favorable strength, hardness (Vickers hardness number around 220), elasticity, corrosion resistance, and accurate with comparatively low cost.

Root Cap Design

The root cap has to meet conventional requirements for root copings:

- preserve the teeth structures from stresses and reinforce them;
- good marginal fit;
- adequate hygiene;
- surface preventing accumulation of plaque;
- non-toxic and compatible with other dental materials;
- corrosion resistant;
- low wear.

Laboratory technique of fabricating a root cap for overdenture retained by magnetic attachments involves specific steps. Firstly, due to the different nature of retention provided by magnetic attachments and, secondly, due to different magnetic attachment materials. Root caps with keeper have several distinct design characteristics:

- small vertical dimension;
- flat surface with no undercuts;
- taper depending on level of bracing required;
- lower requirements for parallelism when several attachments are used;
- applicable with abutments having diminished support.

Root cap has a direct contact with oral environment and the margin of restoration is sometimes located below gingival margin. Moreover coverage of abutments by denture base results in higher plaque accumulation rates, changes in micro-flora composition and subsequently higher risk of periodontal and/or carious lesions. During fabrication of root cap these points have to be kept in mind what will result in restorations and adequately protect abutment teeth.

Working Models and Dies with Silicone Gum Imitation

Similar to the impression quality, the cast and die quality will have a strong effect on accuracy of final restoration. As the margin of restoration is in close proximity to gingival tissues and the whole restoration is covered by the denture base, the marginal architecture and compliance with gingival tissues are of utmost importance.

Prior to pouring a model, surface of impression has to be inspected for clearance. Surface of impression can be sprayed with surfactant in order to increase wetting by dental stone and diminish formation of bubbles. High-strength dental stone (according to ADA, type IV) is commonly used for working models. The impression can be poured accurately just from the first pour-

Fig3 Making index from laboratory putty silicone on working model. It is better to make separate indexes if abutments are located away from each other.

Fig4 Die trimming. A few millimeters area must be removed in order to make space for silicone gum.

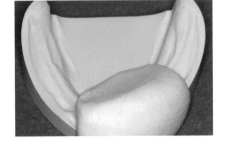
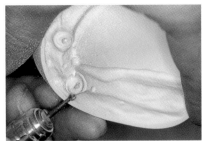

3 | 4

5 | 6

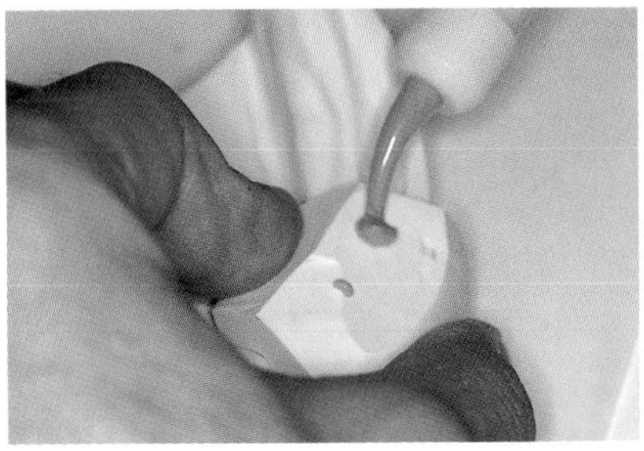

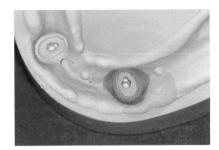

Fig5 Injection of silicone with syringe. It is important to see the excess of silicone coming out from another vent on the index.

Fig6 Completed silicone gum model.

ing and subsequent pouring will result in dimensional changes. Therefore the first pouring has to be done with caution. To avoid bubble formation the vacuum mixing and pouring on vibrating table are recommended. The pouring is started from the most critical area - margin of preparation. Later other small amounts of stone are added incrementally in one place. When the critical areas are completed, larger amounts of stone can be added with the minimal thickness of 5 mm from gingival margin. Following setting the parts where separation will be required are coated with separating agent while parts where separation is not desired are roughened by adding stone blobs. Later the dental stone of contrasting colour is poured leaving the tips of dowel pins uncovered. After the stone sets the cast is trimmed.

Gingiva modelling on the cast is beneficial as it allows visualisation of gingival tissues and better margin adaptation. Firstly the index from putty silicone material (e.g. Lab Silicone, Shofu Japan) in area of abutment is made (Fig3). It is better to make separate indexes if the abutments are located away from each other. The saw cut positions on the cast are marked and the cast is cut just through the first layer of stone without cutting second one. A few millimetres just adjacent to the margin are trimmed away with a round bur to use of microscope in this step is recommended (Fig4). After, isolation, the material is applied with a brush closely to the prepared margin where the stone was trimmed away and to the inner surface of the index. The index is placed over the abutment and through the hole, a gingiva modelling material (e.g. Vestogum, 3M Espe) is injected (Fig5). After setting of the material, the index is removed and gingiva model is finished (Fig6).

Before Making Wax Pattern

The practitioner must understand that every defect or void in the wax will appear in the casting. Most defects can be corrected easily in wax, but not in a metal casting. Careful evaluation of the pattern, preferably under magnification, is critical in obtaining a good casting.

Inlay wax is usually used in fabrication of wax patterns for root caps. The type II inlay waxes are soft and suitable for preparing replicas on dies and models. Wax pattern can undergo considerable distortion easily thus special measures to cope with it should be taken. Therefore the pattern should be invested immediately after the pattern is finished. Before starting wax-up, dies have to be inspected thoroughly. Attention is paid to any bubbles and voids, which can reflect

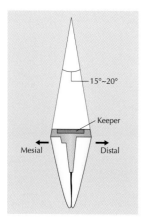

Fig 7 Taper angle of axial walls. It should be 10-15º.

defects of the impressions. In this step all undercuts have to be identified and blocked out (if they are not in proximity of margin). In order to remove the wax pattern from the die easily with application of minimal distortion force, two layers of die lubricant agent applied. Thickness of spacer inside the root canal is virtually impossible to control, thus it can be applied on all surfaces except the root canal. Also it does not cover margin area, where 1 mm is left free of spacer. Thickness of the space provided is recommended 20-40 μm. The margins of root cap are marked with a pencil. Color contrasting to die is preferable as it is more visible and allows better adaptation of the margin. Graphite pencils should be avoided as it can act as an antiflux and cause casting defects at the margin area. Electronic waxing instruments allow better control of temperature and unlike to ordinary waxing instruments they do not contaminate wax pattern with carbon.

Waxing-up before setting Keeper or Housing Pattern

Initially, heated paraffin wax is pressed over the die to achieve good adaptation of wax to root canal walls. Wax has some elasticity and if not heated enough later it can regain its shape and cause distortion. After assurance that post part is well adapted and is of sufficient length, small portions of molten wax are added on the occlusal surface. With adding new portion of wax it has

to be made sure that previously added portion became cool. That helps to control distortion. After proximal surfaces are built up, wax pattern is trimmed at the marginal area. Marginal fit is rechecked on the die with gingival model. If the wax pattern is going to be very thin at the marginal area it can be made thicker during waxing in order to avoid casting defects and adapted latter during finishing and polishing procedures. The vertical height of wax pattern is crucial. The height of the root cap is ruled by vertical interarch space available. It is also determined by the ability of abutment tooth to tolerate stress as higher root cap produces higher levering forces. Roughly the distance from the top of the root cap to the opposing teeth or prothesis should remain as minimum as 3 mm in anterior and 4 mm in posterior region. If abutment teeth are of compromised periodontal condition, the root cap should have lower profile. Finally the axial walls of the wax pattern have to be tapered. The angle of taper plays important role in retention and stability as well as the height. The smaller angle of taper the better retention and stability is achieved. Method of telescope crown is very technique sensitive and is rarely combined with magnetic attachments. Commonly the taper angle is made of around 15° (Fig 7).

Further fabrication of wax pattern differs according to which cast-bonded or cement-bonded keeper technique is going to be used.

Cast-bonded Keeper Technique

Placing keeper in the wax pattern, minimum 0.3 mm thickness of wax should remain between keeper and tooth structures (Fig 8)[3]. This is necessary to ensure proper casting. After determining vertical dimension of root cap the occlusal surface is made flat and as possible parallel to the occlusal plane and other root caps if several magnetic attachments are going to be used (Fig 9).

Fig 8 Thickness of the wax under the keeper. At least 0.3mm is needed.
Fig 9 Occlusal surfaces of root caps before setting keepers. They are flat and almost parallel.

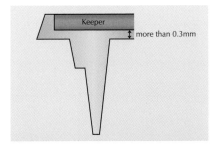

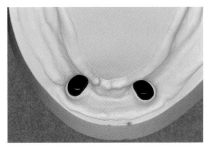

8 | 9

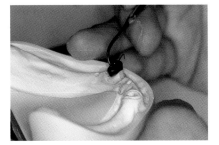

Fig 10 Setting keeper on the wax pattern. It is very important to heat and add enough wax around keeper to achieve good integrity and prevent crevice formation.

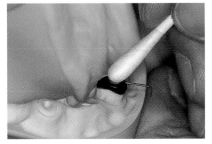

Fig 11 Occlusal surface of the root cap is smoothened with cotton pallet dipped in alcohol.

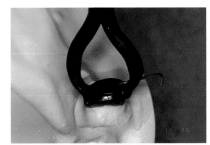

Fig 12 Y-shape sprue attached to the pattern. Such sprue design is highly recommended because of the presence of the keeper.

Keeper Selection

At this point the shape and size of magnetic attachment are confirmed definitely. The roots of anterior teeth have oval shape cross section and the posterior teeth circular. Selecting the shape of magnetic attachment corresponding to the cross-section of root enables more efficient utilization of occlusal surface. The size of keeper is governed by the diameter of the root, and taper angle and height of the root cap. As it is preferable to deliver balanced retention in both sides of the arch, similar size (thus retention) magnetic attachments can be applied on each side if possible. That will aid in denture stability and prevent it from rotational movements during function.

As keepers used with cast-bonded technique have to be somehow fixed in the investment material during casting, they have handles attached to its lateral aspect. This leaves the occlusal surface of keeper intact and aids in better fit of the keeper and magnetic attachment surfaces. As the keeper has to be firmly secured to the investment material the handle prior setting the keeper is bended to prevent rotation.

Keeper Setting

To do this the keeper with bended handle is orientated on the top of the wax pattern. Wax on the occlusal surface is melted and under the control of direction, the keeper is slowly settled into the wax pattern (Fig 10). If more than one keeper are planned it is highly recommended to use keeper setting tool. Keeper setting tool prevents setting of keepers in unparallel manner to the occlusal plane and to each other. However magnetic attachments are not angle sensitive as mechanical ones, and only considerably unparallel keepers may have clinical difficulties. If the angulation of abutment teeth permits, parallel setting of keepers will yield maximum retention of the overdenture.

When the proper position and alignment of keepers are confirmed, the wax pattern is finished. Residual wax around the keeper in occlusal surface should be removed. Thus the surface is smoothened again with waxing instrument and finally polished with alcohol-dipped cotton pallet (Fig 11).

Spruing

The metal flow during casting is disturbed by

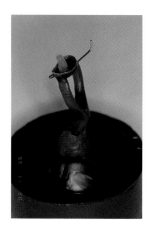

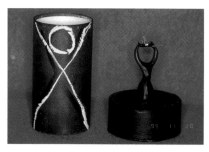

13 | 14

Fig 13 Wax pattern mounted on sprue-crucible former.
Fig 14 Wax pattern on the crucible former and ring. It should be located above the center of the ring where the temperature is highest and can result casting voids.

the presence of the keeper. It is of great importance to ensure proper metal flow around the perimeter of the keeper, otherwise the keeper will be poorly attached to the root cap and the presence of crevice will dramatically cause corrosion and discolouration. Therefore it is highly recommended to use Y-shape double sprues and attach them to the opposite sides of the wax pattern. The sprue must be large enough so that it remains open until the casting solidifies and short enough to allow rapid filling of the mold cavity. For casting root cap, a sprue of 1,5 mm in diameter and 4-5 mm in length will fulfil these requirements. The sprues are made of curved wax wires and joined at the top of the plastic former (*Fig 12*). Sprues should be attached at the bulkiest portion of the wax pattern and cannot be located close to the margin as it will impinge on marginal fit.

Investment and Casting

It is advised to readapt the margins of the pattern immediately before investment since it can be distorted due to elasticity of the wax or other factors. The wax pattern is mounted on the sprue pin, which in turn is mounted on a clean sprue-crucible-former base (*Fig 13*). The wax pattern has to be at around 6 mm from the end of the ring as it is considered as the optimal distance allowing diffusion of gases and preventing the investment from braking during casting. Also the wax pattern can't be located at the center of the

ring where the alloy solidifies lastly and resulting in porosity of it (*Fig 14*). Gypsum-bonded investment materials are used with type IV gold alloys. Before investing it is made sure that the keeper handle protrudes sufficiently (minimum 3 mm) and is bent. Then surfactants for improving wetting of wax pattern are sprayed. The initial amount of the investment material is applied with brush without the ring placed on the former base. After assuring the coverage of whole pattern's surface by investment material, the ring is placed on the base and filled by investment material. After setting of investment, the mold is placed in the furnace at 700ºC for burning out the wax for about 1 hour. It is recommended to keep the mold in the furnace 15 min longer than usual. The prolonged burnout aids elevation of keeper's temperature and improving the casting along the borders of the keeper. On the other hand overheating of keeper as it was mentioned can cause oxidization. Therefore the temperature higher than 700ºC should be avoided. After casting, the mold ring is left for the bench cooling until its temperature reaches the room temperature. It is not advised to immerse the ring into cold water immediately after casting because the crevice between keeper and metal cap alloy can increase and results in loosing hardness of the alloy.

Divesting and Pickling

Divesting is accomplished by hand instruments and sandblasting. The cleaned casting has

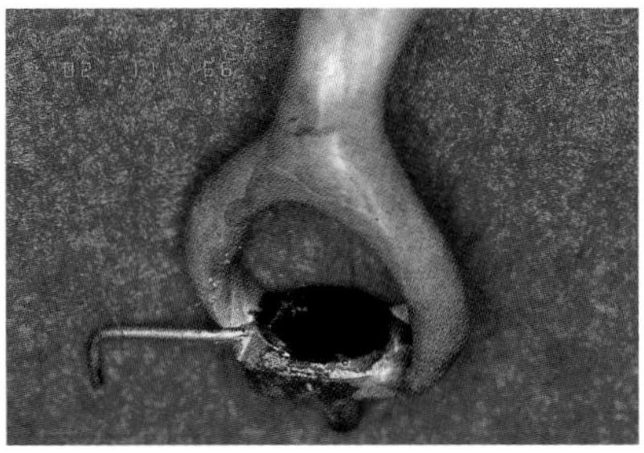

Fig 15 Divested and sandblasted casting before finishing and polishing. The surface is covered with oxide film.
Fig 16 Pickling unit and solution to remove the oxide film. The keeper is sensitive to acids. Its surface should be covered with petroleum or cyanoacrylate glue.

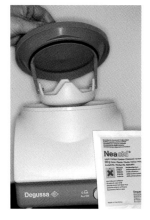
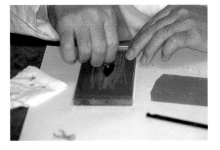
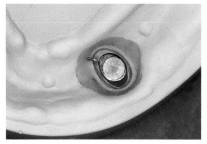

Fig 17 Rouge varnished water-polishing paper (#2000) on glass plate. The surface of the keeper is polished by hand using one direction movement.
Fig 18 Finished and polished root cap with keeper on the working model.

a dark and tarnished color (*Fig 15*) owing to oxide or sulfide deposits. They are removed by placing the casting in a pickling solution (*Fig 16*). Such a solution is usually an acid or a combination of acids with an HCl base. The ferromagnetic stainless steel of keeper is very sensitive to acids, hence the pickling solution is carefully selected and high temperature pickling is not recommended. Before pickling the surface of the keeper is covered by petroleum or cyanoacrylate glue in order to protect it. If the color of the solution is changed it has to be replaced. Metal tongs cannot be used as well. After pickling castings are rinsed with water.

Finishing and Polishing

The precision of fit and marginal integrity is checked on the die and if the casting was done properly, only minor corrections are needed. After the root cap has been set it is finished with silicone rubber, rag or felt wheels impregnated with abrasives. Care should be exercised not to touch the keeper surface. Root cap can be polished by various oxides of tin and aluminum used in conjunction with a small rag, followed

with iron oxide rouge. Polishing of the occlusal surface of the root cap is a critical step. As the performance of magnetic attachment is highly influenced by quality of contact between the keeper and magnetic assembly, occlusal surface of the root cap containing the keeper have to be smooth, plane and without scratches. Therefore the water-polishing paper (advised roughness index #2000) is placed on a glass plate - to ensure smooth surface - and the surface of it is rubbed with rouge. This reduces abrasiveness of the paper and increase polishing properties. Then by holding post, the root cap is placed on the polishing paper and the occlusal surface is rubbed several times carefully (*Fig 17*). After polishing, the root cap with keeper is set on the model and delivered in the dental clinic for intraoral fitting and cementation (*Fig 18*).

Cement-bonded Keeper Technique[4]

Another way of attaching keeper to the root cap is cement-bonded keeper technique. Unlike cast-bonded technique, the root cap is cast without keeper. The keeper is attached to the root cap by means of adhesive cement after root cap cast-

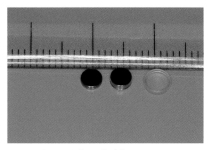 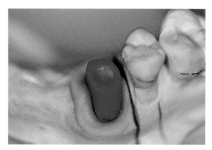 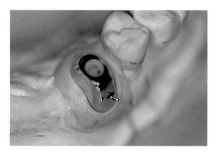

Fig 19 Cement-bonded keeper, magnetic assembly and housing pattern. Housing pattern is 0.1-0.2 mm larger than keeper in order to leave space for adhesive cement.

Fig 20 Wax pattern on die with silicone gum removed. The top of the housing pattern should be in the same level with wax in occlusal surface.

Fig 21 Polished root cap on the working model with silicone gum. The keeper is not cemented yet.

ing, finishing and polishing. The cement-bonded keeper technique is quite similar to the cast-bonded technique.

First of all, the magnetic attachment is selected according to the available area of the root cross-section, shape of it and prospective design of the root cap. Similarly, a minimum of 0.3 mm of metal around the keeper is required. Magnetic attachments compatible with cement-bonded technique have specially designed housing patterns that ensure appropriate space for keeper and bonding agent (Fig 19). The wax pattern of the root cap is made in the same way as with cast-bonded technique. Then the occlusal surface of the wax pattern is softened with hot waxing instrument and housing pattern is inserted into the softened wax. If several magnetic attachments are planed the assistance of setting tools is recommended. It should be ascertained that housing pattern is placed in the same level with occlusal surface of wax pattern (this is made to allow finishing and polishing of the root cap). The excess of wax is trimmed away and contours of the wax pattern re-established. The wax pattern is polished prior to casting, as it will make the finishing and polishing of the root cap much easier (Fig 20).

Wax pattern is sprued as an ordinary root coping. Use of Y-shaped sprue design is not necessary. Still the sprue has to be of 1.5 mm in diameter and 4-5 mm in length, and attached to the bulkiest portion of the wax pattern and located somehow between the margin of the root cap and the housing pattern. If there is no choice the proximity to housing pattern is selected. Investment, burnout and casting procedures are done following manufacturers recommendations.

Divesting, pickling, finishing and polishing are carried out after then. In contrast to cast-bonded technique pickling as well as finishing and polishing can be done without damaging the keeper. The inner part of the housing where the keeper will be located is not finished or polished. The occlusal surface of the root cap is made as smooth as possible and final polishing on a glass plate with water-polishing paper is recommended. This will ensure close contact of the keeper and the magnet assembly. After polishing, the root cap is re-seated on the die and the keeper is cemented before delivey in dental clinic (Fig 21).

Cementation of the Keeper

Adhesive cements are very technique sensitive, so it is important how handy particular type of cement is with clinician. Due to its biocompatibility and good adhesion to the metal, Super-Bond C&B (SunMedical, Japan) is suitable for cementation of the keeper and/or the root cap as well. Prior to cementation, the keeper is fitted to the root cap. The occlusal surface of the keeper should be in the same plane with occlusal surface of root cap. The surface of root cap and keeper are roughened by sandblasting. Care should be taken not to sandblast the polished surfaces of the root cap and occlusal surface of the keeper.

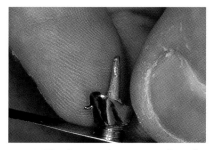

Fig 22 The keeper is cemented to the root cap.

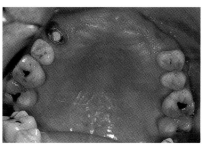

Fig 23 Root cap with cement-bonded keeper in situ.

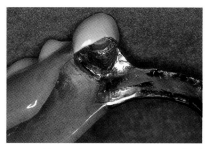

Fig 24 Magnetic overdenture repaired with custom made metal artificial tooth. Magnetic assembly is cement-bonded to crown. Artificial tooth was changed because of fracture of resin tooth.

Table 1: Comparison between cast- and cement-bonded keepers.

Issue	Cast-bonded keeper technique	Cement-bonded keeper technique
Spruing	Two sprues recommended	One sprue at bulkiest portion is adequate
Casting	Possibility of casting defects if spruing and preheating is not adequate	Easy
Pickling	Protection of keeper by appropriate pickling regime and covering by petroleum is assured	According to manufacturer instructions
Polishing	Care exercised not to roughen surface of keeper	Smoothness of keeper is guaranteed as keeper is cemented after polishing root cap
Crevice corrosion	Possible if casting defects in cast-keeper interface are present or keeper is overheated	Possible if cement loss around keeper appears
Cementation of keeper	–	Technique sensitive
Orientation of keeper	Secured during casting	Can undergo slight dislocation during cementation

The keeper is then placed on a spatula with occlusal surface facing it, the adhesive resin is applied on roughened surfaces of the keeper and root cap. The root cap is placed over the keeper on the spatula (Fig 22). The use of cement in abundance should be avoided as it can interfere with proper contact of root cap and the surface of spatula and consequently the keeper will be cemented in a wrong position. After setting, the excess of cement is removed and occlusal surface of the root cap is polished (Fig 23).

Versatile Usage of Housing Patterns

Similarly as for making space for the keeper in the root cap, special housing patterns can be employed for making space for magnetic assembly in metal overdenture base or cast crown (Fig 24). This technique can be useful in clinical situations when vertical space is limited and does not permit adequate thickness of acrylic base or "metal-touch" design.

Comparison of Cast-bonded and Cement-bonded Keeper Techniques

Although both techniques if done properly assure long-term service of restorations, there are several differences which have to be considered. They are summarized in Table 1.

References

1. Mizutani H, Nakamura K, Ai M: Influence of Thermal Cycle on Attractive Force of Magnetic Attachment. J Dent Res 74 (Special Issue): 471, 1995.

2. Okuno O, Takada Y, Kinouchi Y, Mizutani H, Ai M, Yamada H : Corrosion Resistance of Magnetic Stainless Steel for Magnetic Attav\chment. J Dent Res 74 (Special Issue): 559, 1995.

3. Mizutani H, Ishihata N, Nakamura K, Ai M: Tooth Preparation and Laboratory Procedure. Removable Partial Denture Used with Magnetic Attachment. 43–48, Tokyo, Quintessence Publishing. 1994.

4. Mizutani H: Reconsiderations of Magnetic Attachments in the Field of Removable Partial Prosthodontics – A Process to Heatless Keeper-. Program of the 6th Meeting International research Project of Magnetic Dentistry, 2002.

Chapter 10

The Root Keeper System and its clinical application

Yuh-Yuan Shiau

How the Root Keeper System was Developed

Using magnet to retain a denture on the alveolar ridge had long been considered (Ai, 1994; Gillings, 1981). Many designs had been proposed and clinically applied (Laird et al, 1981). However, because of the corrosion (Drago,1981) and biological effects of the magnetic materials (Atlay et al, 1991) and the size required to provide sufficient attraction force, those designs proposed before 1980s were not satisfactory and long lasted (Riley et al, 2001). It was Dr. Gillings who introduced the newly developed rare-earth magnetic materials and the concept of magnet-keeper system that magnetic attachment regained its reputation and has been clinically accepted (Gillings, 1981; Gillings, 1983). Since then, the magnet is no longer inserted on the root, but is adhered to the denture side, thus reduced the biological effects of the magnet in the oral cavity (Kawata et al, 1981; Donnohue et al, 1995). The increase of the magnetic attraction force with the decrease of the magnet size has been continuously improved on both the magnetic material selection and the way to house such material (Highton et al, 1986; Jonkman et al, 1995). The keeper part was firstly adhered to the root surface of the abutment tooth with luting agents currently used to cement the crown or inlay onto the tooth (Moghadam and Skandrett, 1979; Gillings, 1984). The durability and strength of those cements were not sufficient that the keepers were often detached and the root surface became carious. The cast post and root cap with the keeper was then proposed (Smith et al, 1983). The marginal gap between the cap and root surface can be minimized through careful impression and casting, and the risk of caries formation and cement resolve after long-term use is also minimized.

The demand of impression taking, model pouring, investing, and casting for cast keeper fabrication is relatively time wasting and technique dependant. More visits of the patient are required, and the satisfactory keeper part can be obtained only after meticulous laboratory procedures by a skillful technician. The hope of inserting the keeper with a prefabricated post directly at chair-side was raised again when the resin cement was introduced and its durability and strength were highly appreciated.

Moreover, when a patient with magnetic keeper in a root requires magnetic resonance imaging (MRI) examination of the cranium, the keeper will often cause an interference of the magnetic field, and a dark shadow is formed. The keeper should be removed if the interference is to be eliminated. However, the cast post and root cap with the keeper are not easy to be removed without hurting the root structure. Retrievable keeper is required when removal of the keeper is necessary and resetting of the keeper later on is also necessary. Based on at least the above reasons, the manufacturers of the magnetic attachments were asked to develop cementing type

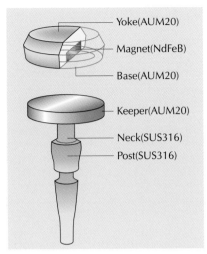

- Yoke(AUM20)
- Magnet(NdFeB)
- Base(AUM20)
- Keeper(AUM20)
- Neck(SUS316)
- Post(SUS316)

Fig 1 Components of a typical RK system

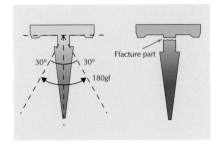

30° 30°
180gf
Ffacture part

Fig 2 Maximum bending angle and force of a RK keeper

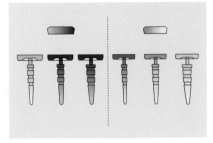

Fig 3 Types of the RK system.
Left side : L type, diameter = 4.0mm; thickness of the magnet = 1.3mm; thickness of the keepr = 0.8mm.
Right side : S type, diameter = 3.6mm; thickness of the magnet = 1.1mm; thickness of the keepr = 0.7mm.
The diameter of the post varied from 1.0mm to 1.5mm in both L and S types.

keeper for wider clinical use.

On the magnet part, disc type magnet was developed before the sandwich yoke system was developed. Magfit system for example, has its magnetic material housed in a rectangular yoke which has better corrosion and abrasion resistance. However, it was found that disc type magnet can produce more powerful magnetic force with minimized size than the sandwich type magnet. The Root Keeper system was thus developed because of the demand of powerful and small magnets.

What is the Root Keeper System?

The Root Keeper System (RK system) was developed and produced by the Aichi Steel Co. Japan in year 2000. It was firstly used in Japan and then in Taiwan and Korea. Although the name of this system "Root Keeper" is often confused with the term "root keepers" used to describe the keeper part on the root (Riley et al, 1999), the RK system still obtained its reputation because of its convenience in use. The system comprises a disc type magnetic assembly and a disc type keeper with a post (Fig 1). The keeper part is made of AUM20, a magnetizable stainless steel and the post is made of SUS316, a non-magnetic stainless steel. These two parts are laser

welded without solder material. The magnetic assembly is a disc-shaped yoke of AUM20, which houses a rare-earth magnetic material (Nd-Fe-B alloy) (Okuno et al, 1989). The base of the magnetic assembly is covered by a thin layer of AUM20, which is sealed to the yoke with laser welding. Two sizes of the discs are provided, i.e.4.0mm and 3.6mm in diameter with two sizes of posts, i.e. 1.5mm and 1.0mm in diameter. The length of the post is 7.0mm. The thickness of the keeper is 0.7 or 0.8mm and that of the magnetic assembly is 1.1mm and 1.3 mm. Therefore the total thickness of the magnet-keeper assembly is 1.8mm at least and 2.1mm at most. There is a relatively thinner part of the post approximating the base of the keeper, and that is the part to be bended. The maximum bending angle and force are suggested to be 30 degrees and 180gf (Fig 2). One to three serrated cuts were provided on the shaft of the post for better post retention. Diagrammatic figures of the system can be seen more in details at Fig 3.

During cementation, a dual-cure composite resin cement is recommended. Light cure resin should not be used because the light is unable to reach the root part cement. For better adhesion, the surface of the post and the base of the keeper should be covered with 4-META resin and illu-

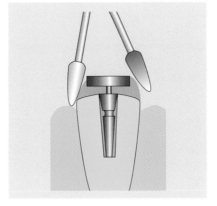

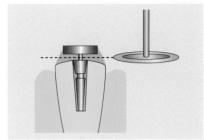

Fig 4 Inserted RK keeper with composite resin. The resin surface should be trimmed and polished with green and white stones.
Fig 5 The cemented keeper can be removed by cutting the neck with a carborundum dics.

4 | 5

minated. When the composite resin is set, the exposed resin surface surrounding the keeper should be trimmed and smoothened (Fig 4).

Indications for the Use of the RK System

The RK system can be used on any cases which are indicated for magnetic attachment retained partial dentures or overdentures. However, some conditions are more suitable for the use of the RK system.

1. Handicapped patients with difficulties in handling their dentures: A conventional removable partial denture requires clasps on the abutment teeth to obtain its retention and stability. Moreover, a retentive clasp has a tapered distal arm, which is fit properly on the abutment tooth without a gap. A patient with awkward hand or finger movement has difficulties to remove such clasps. The patients are then refrained from withdrawing their denture thus resulted in poor oral hygiene and then dental caries and periodontitis. Reduction of the abutment height after intention endodontic treatment and then insertion of the RK system can prevent further periodontal destruction and avoid awkwardness on denture withdrawal.

   Furthermore, because the cemented root keeper of the RK system has minimum root cap height, there is minimum prevention of lateral displacement compare with Magfit system and other mechanical attachment systems used for

denture prosthesis. Therefore, the handicapped patients can withdraw the denture by just holding the denture flange and exert a lateral force with ease.

2. In now a day medical care point of view, MRI examination is more often prescribed. When MRI of head and neck is indicated, removal of the magnetic devices in the oral cavity is necessary. Removal of the keeper from the root is easier than the cast keeper assembly because the neck of keeper is thin and the root surface is covered with composite resin (Fig 5). The risk of damaging the root structure and the keeper is minimum. Reinsert a new keeper is also easy by trimming away some composite resin on the root and insert a new keeper without a post with appropriate resin cement.

3. Patients who have limited time for dental treatment or have to complete treatment in one visit: Cast root cap with keeper for magnetic attachment denture prosthesis requires more than one visit after the completion of endodontic treatment. The cast keeper prosthesis requires impression and casting in the dental lab and the patient may not have sufficient time to wait or come again to obtain such treatment. If the RK system is used, insertion of a keeper-post with resin cement and then installation of a new denture tooth with a magnet on the re-contoured denture base over the root and keeper can be done in one visit. The so constructed denture can be

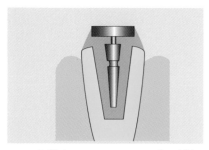

Fig6 Sufficient cement space should be provided in order not to cause wedging effect of the post during insertion.

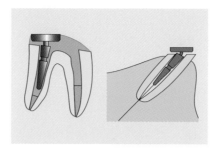

Fig7 Non-axial occlusal load can be obtained by changing the keeper-post angle.

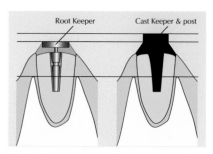

Fig8 Comparison of root cap height between RK system and cast keeper-post system.

served as an interim denture or definite one for a long period of use.

4. Seriously deteriorated root surface due to caries or fracture: After removal of the decayed or destructed tissues, the root surface may become irregular with undercuts. Impression and waxing of the root cap with a keeper is more difficult. In such cases, insertion of a keeper with composite resin under direct visual approach has better chance to obtain a complete coverage of the irregular root surface. Moreover, the root canal may have been enlarged during root canal instrumentation and the remaining dental structure may become weak. Insertion of a cast root cap with a snugly fit post may often cause fracture of the root during cementation. The RK post is prefabricated and its size and length can be selected to provide sufficient space for cement without causing wedging effect during cementation (Fig6). In addition, the resin cement may shrink during setting and pull the surrounding dental structure together instead of forcing it apart.

5. Abutment root with non-parallel axis to the denture path of insertion: Quite often the root canal of a retained root is not parallel to the path of denture insertion. If a cast post with a keeper is not parallel to that path, retention force of the magnetic attachment would be reduced. The RK system provides the user a maximum of 30° changing allowance, the keeper can have better chance to meet the

magnet at right angle (Fig7).

6. Insufficient edentulous space for denture prosthesis: Since the total thickness of the RK keeper and root cap is much less than the Magfit system and other attachment systems, the RK system has better chance to provide denture support in patients with insufficient interalveolar space(Fig8). Furthermore, patients who have limited mouth opening ability often do not allow proper impression needed for cast restorations. The RK system can then be used for such patients if denture prosthesis is needed or a denture is to be repaired.

7. For better anterior esthetics of an overdenture: Overdentures rest on anterior roots may often result in thinning of the denture base at that area. If the roots are covered with metal root-caps, the dark color of the metal may be seen much easier. The root cap of the RK system comprises a metal keeper and composite resin collar, thus, the metallic shadow is not as evident.

Special Care for the Use of the RK System

1. Since the RK keeper has the advantage of easily removable if necessary, the keeper should not be inserted too close to the root surface. A space of about 1.0-2.0mm above the top of the root should be provided (Fig9).

2. The post of the RK keeper should not be snugly fitting to the root canal. The post

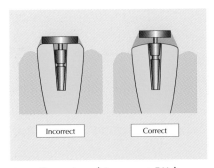

Fig 9 Correct and incorrect RK keeper position in a prepared root. Sufficient cement should be presented between the keeper and the root.

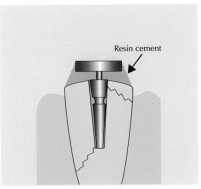

Fig 10 Fracture of the root may happen if the post is snugly fitting the root.

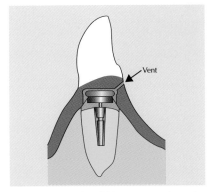

Fig 11 A vent should be prepared on the denture base close to the magnetic attachment system to assure the filling of resin and maintain the right position of the magnet.

should be loosely embedded in the canal with sufficient space for the luting cement, otherwise fracture of the root may happen during keeper insertion or after use (*Fig 10*).

3. The composite resin surrounding the keeper should be trimmed carefully without leaving an overhang over the root margin. Most of the gingival inflammation condition is caused by the irritating effect of the overhang resin. Finishing and polishing of the resin surface should also be thorough.

Possible Risks of using the RK System

The advantages of using the RK system mentioned above provided clinicians an alternative of attachment retained partial dentures. However, some risks are predictable, and should be avoided.

1. Gingival inflammation of the abutment root: This is the most common pathological change found in magnetic attachment retained denture. Careless forming of the resin root cap with overhang margin is the main reason of such change. Besides, because the root-cap of the RK system is short, the risk of impinging the surrounding gingival tissue is more possible. Careful elimination of the denture acrylic resin surrounding the root surface is necessary.

2. Detachment of the keeper: Because of the destructed resin and the fracture of the neck part of the keeper, the keeper may become detached (Wigianto and Kusumadewi, 2002). Fortunately, the detached keeper is often retained on the magnet in the denture thus the patient can find that keeper without the worry of swallowing the keeper. Replacement of a new keeper is easy. The operator can either trim away the resin and remove the post and then replace with a new keeper-post or just leave the post in the canal and then replace with a keeper without the post. Care must be taken to meet the magnet at right position. If the position of a new keeper does not meet the magnet properly, reposition of the magnet in the denture base is necessary.

3. Fracture or wear of the resin after long term use: The exposed resin collar on the root may not be strong enough to resist compression and impact force during chewing and clenching. Fracture or wear of the resin may then happen, and the formation of root caries and gingival inflammation is possible. Careful self-inspection and routine recall at least every 6 months are recommended to reveal such defects earlier. Replacement of new resin is easy if the keeper remains intact.

4. Miscellaneous: Corrosion of the magnetic assembly due to breakage of the yoke may happen after long term use or careless cuts on the magnet assembly (Shiau and Liu,1998).

Loss of magnetic retention force is the first sign of such defect. A magnetic sensor can be used for magnetic force detection. Replacement of the decayed magnet with a new one is of ten necessary after years of overdenture use (Van Waas et al, 1996). Replacement of a new magnet is easy and should be done about 2 years after insertion.

In general, the RK system can be categorized as an alternative of attachment denture treatment modalities. Careful selection of cases is the key to success. Although a periodontally compromised abutment root can still be used as RK abutment, a subgingival root or root with very thin remaining structure should not be used. Careful handling of the thin magnet is necessary. Because the magnet is thin, the retention of it in the denture base requires operator's skilful hands and proper application of the self-cure acrylic resin. Provision of a vent in the denture base during magnet pick up is a good way to assure the right positioning of the magnet in the denture base (*Fig 11*). Recent products of the RK magnet provided resin coating on its top surfaces, thus helped the adhesion of the denture base resin. Last but not least, patient's thorough home care and regular recalls with professional care are necessary to prevent the loss of periodontal support due to chronic inflammation.

Clinical Application of Root Keeper System

Case 1

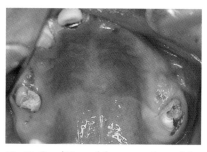

Fig 12 Condition of the upper jaw of the patient.

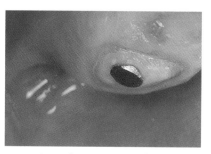

Fig 13 A root keeper was applied on 27.

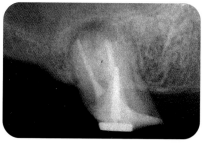

Fig 14 A root keeper applied to the distal root of 27.

15 | 16

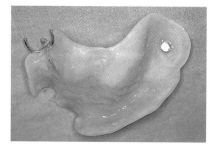

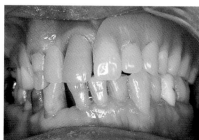

Fig 15 A magnet fixed to the denture.
Fig 16 The denture set in the mouth.

Male, 62 years old, had poor oral hygiene because of mental retardation and poor communication. His denture was supported by 27 and 16 with conventional clasps. 27 became carious and painful and its pulp was extirpated (*Fig 12*). A root keeper was applied on the distal root with composite resin (*Fig 13, 14*). A new resin tooth was added and the denture base repaired (*Fig 15, 16*). The patient was encouraged to take off and clean his denture after meals with just a simple lateral and downward pull of the denture.

Case 2

Fig 17 A root keeper was applied to 44. Magnet is on the keeper.
Fig 18 A new artificial tooth was added to the denture.

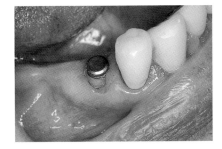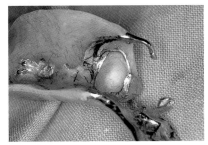

17 | 18

Fig 19 A magnet was fixed to the denture.
Fig 20 The denture set in the mouth.

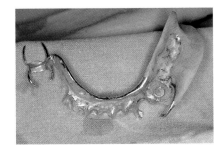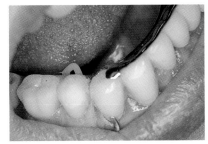

19 | 20

Female, 52 years old, had a partial denture using 35, 36, 43 as abutments. 44 was not in good shape and was not used at very beginning. One year later, 44 became mobile and painful, and endodontic treatment was done under the consideration that the root of 44 could help the stability of the denture. Because of the poor bony support of 44, lateral stress should be avoided. A RK system was applied and a new denture tooth was added (Fig 17, 18). The magnetic attachment helped the clasp to retain and stabilize the denture with satisfactory outcomes (Fig 19, 20).

Case 3

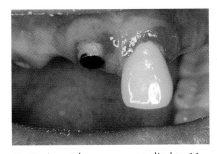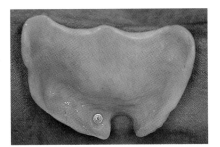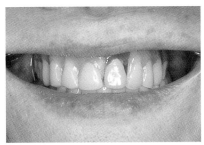

Fig 21 A root keeper was applied to 11.

Fig 22 A magnet was fixed to the denture.

Fig 23 The denture set in the mouth.

Female, 65 years old, had systemic diabetic problem and arthritis for decades. Her oral hygiene was poor and her gingival tissues were always at inflammatory condition because of her diabetes mellitus and arthritic hands. She had two remaining teeth on the upper jaw to support her ill-fitting upper partial denture. 11 was then endodontically treated because of deep caries and pulpitis. RK magnetic attachment was applied on it because of her time limit and awkward finger movement (Fig 23). A new denture tooth was added and the denture base repaired (Fig 21, 22). Three months after this, her 21 was also cut and another RK magnet was applied.

References

1. Ai M : The use of magnetic attachment on removable partial denture. Quintessence publishing, Tokyo, Chap9: 65–71, 1994.

2. Altay O T, Kutkam T, Koseoglu O, Tanyeri S : The biological effects of implanted magnetic fields on the bone tissue of dogs. Int J Oral Maxillofac Implants, 6: 345–349, 1991.

3. Drago C J : Tarnish and corrosion with the use of intra-oral magnets. J Prosthet Dent 66: 536–540, 1981.

4. Gillings B R : Magnetic retention for complete and partial overdentures. Part I. J Prosthet Dent, 45: 484–491, 1981.

5. Gillings B R : Magnetic retention for overdentures. Part II. J Prosthet Dent , 49: 607–618, 1983.

6. Highton R, Caputo A A, Matyas J : Retentive and stress characteristics for a magnetically retained partial overdenture. J Oral Rehabil, 13: 443–450, 1986.

7. Jonkman R E, Van Waas M A, Kalk W : Satisfaction with complete intermediate dentures and complete intermediate overdentures: A 1-year study. J Oral Rehabil, 22: 791–796, 1995.

8. Kawata Y, Shiota H, Tsutsui Y, Yoshida H, Kinouchi Y: Cytotoxicity of Pd-Co dental casting ferromagnetic alloys. J Dent Res, 60: 1403–1409, 1981.

9. Laird W R, Grant A A, Smith G A : The use of magnetic forces in prosthetic dentistry. J Dent, 9: 328–335, 1981.

10. Moghadam B K, Scadrett F R : Magnetic retention for overdentures J Prosthet Dent, 41: 26–29, 1979.

11. Okuno O, Nakano T, Hamanaka H, Kinouchi Y : Encapsulated sandwich type dental magnetic retainers by NdFeB magnet and permandur yoke. Proceedings of the 10th International Workshop on Rare Earth Magnets and Applications, Japan, 1989.

12. Riley M A, Williams A J, Speight J D, Wamsley A D, Harris I R: Investigations into the failure of dental magnets. Int J prosthodont, 12: 249–254, 1999.

13. Shiau Y Y, Liu C C: Evaluation of the retention form of the Magfit magnetic attachment system. J Japan Magnetic Dentistry, 7: 31–34, 1998.

14. Smith G A, Laird W R, Grant A A : Magnetic retention units for overdentures. J Oral Rehabil, 10: 481–488, 1983.

15. van Waas M A, Kalk W, van Zetten B L, van Os J H: Treatment results with immediate overdentures : An evaluation of 4.5 years. J Prosthet Dent, 76: 153–157, 1996.

16. Wigianto R, Kusumadewi S : Breaking down of Root Keeper System : a case report. 6th International Symposium on Magnetic Dentistry (abstract 13), 2002.

Chapter 11

Clinical Analysis on the Reliability of the Magnetic Attachments over an 8 year period

Hiroshi Inoue

Introduction

In recent years, dimensions of magnets have been considerably reduced without compromising the force of retention, and making such magnets suitable for dental applications. Consequently, magnetic attachments are available for various prosthodontic procedures[1, 2].

However, we encountered several problems over the years when they were utilized in more patients. In this study, problems with dentures and abutment teeth with magnetic attachments observed over 8 years are summarized.

Materials and Methods

Patients treated with magnetic attachments at Osaka Dental University Hospital from November 9, 1992 to August 30, 2000 were included in this analysis. The attachments used were MAGFIT, MAGSOFT and MAGNEDISC (Aichi Steel). The subjects consisted of 30 males and 47 females. There were 85 denture bases and 11 dentures. There were 116 abutment teeth in total. Data were collected from the clinical records completed by the practitioners from November 9, 1992 to November 1, 2000.

Problems with dentures and abutments, and the onset of the problems were examined.

The relationship between the occurrence of problem and time course of it were analyzed by plotting a cumulative survival curve using the Kaplan-Meier method (*Fig 1*). Prognostic factors were classified into two categories which were compared using the Logrank test at a significance level of 0.05. The paired categories were dentists with more than 10 years of clinical experience and those with less than that.

Results and Discussion

The ratio of newly made dentures and repair and modification of the existing denture were shown in *Fig 2*. New denture application accounts for 55 cases, and holds 65% of the share, while repair and accounts for 30 cases, and holds 35%.

The cases involving repair of an existing denture with magnetic attachments accounts for a surprising 35%.

Fig 3 shows the abutments teeth problems, which are 43 in number, accounting for 38% of the total 116 abutment teeth. 16% were extracted, 11%, had keeper separation, 9% fell out, and 2% had carries. *Fig 4* shows the denture problems. 26 or 30.6% of total 85 denture bases, had problems. 21.2% had fractures, 9.4% had magnet separation. 64.9% experienced no problems.

The cumulative survival curve of the dentures is shown in *Fig 5–9*. *Fig 5* is the curve in which the end point is decided when first trouble has occured as magnet separation or fracture of the dentures. The duration of the observation is from 0.5 months of 86.6 months, with the mean value of 25.2 months. The survival rate at the end of the observation period was 57.2%. The slope of the curve is significant until 40 months, at which

Fig 1 What is the Kaplan-Meier method.

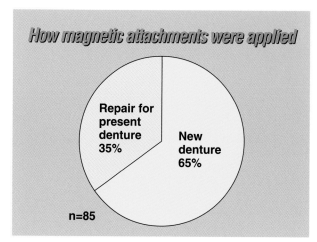

How magnetic attachments were applied

Fig 2 How magnetic attachments were applied.

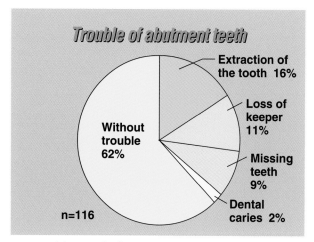

Fig 3 Problems with abutment teeth.

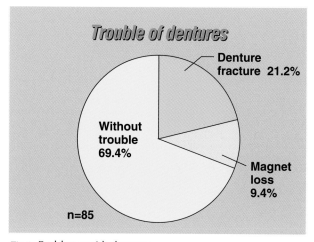

Fig 4 Problems with dentures.

point it levels off. This indicates that denture trouble is likely to occur within 40 months of denture installation.

Fig 6 shows the survival curve when an end point is the loss after denture function. The duration of the observation is from 0.9 months to 86.6 months, with a mean of 29.4 months. The survival rate at the end of the observation period was 97.1%. This high survival rate was possible because dentures were refitted after magnet separation, and repaired after tooth extraction so that they could continue to be used with no problem. These results reflect that how easy the laboratory procedures of magnetic attachments are compared to other retainers, and how easy it is to use in an existing denture.

The cumulative survival curve of abutments is shown in both *Fig 7* and *Fig 8*. *Fig 7* is the curve

in which the endpoint is decided to be keeper separation, caries, extraction, or natural teeth loss. The duration of the observation is from 2.1 months to 85.3 months, with the mean value of 38.9 months. The slope becomes significant at 71 months, and the survival rate becomes zero at 7th year. Generally speaking, using the Kaplan-Meier method, the fluctuation of the survival rate becomes greater in the last part of the observation duration[3]. This is because the population, or the number of cases, becomes smaller due to censored cases, and the survival rates are inferred from fewer number of cases.

Fig 8 shows the curve when an end point is decided a "when the abutment cannot be used anymore". The observation duration is from 2.1 months to 86.6 months, with a mean value of 39.0 months. The survival rate at the end was

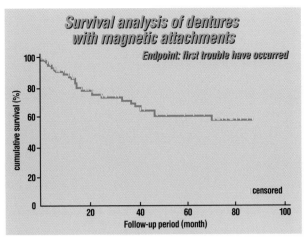

Fig 5 Survival analysis of dentures with magnetic attachment. Endpoint : onset of first problem.

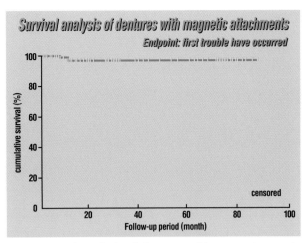

Fig 6 Survival analysis of dentures with magnetic attachment. Endpoint : the loss of dentre function.

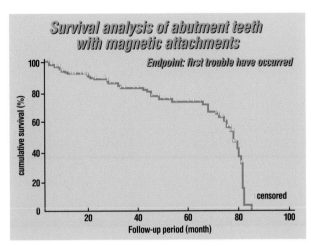

Fig 7 Survival analysis of abutment teeth with magnetic attachments. Endpoint : one set of first problem.

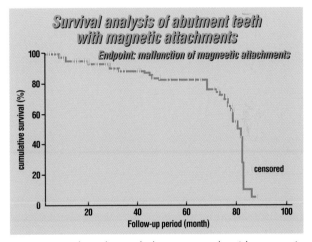

Fig 8 Survival analysis of abutment teeth with magnetic attachments. Endpoint : malfunction of magnetic attachment.

5.6%. When keeper separation was observed, it was repaired and functioned well afterwards or at I mentioned earlier. However, more than half of the troubles were extraction and natural teeth loss. This may be the reason that there is not much difference between *Fig 7* and *Fig 8*, even though there is some difference at the end survival rates.

Fig 9 shows the curve for the separation of the magnet from the denture base. There is a significant difference between groups, and experienced dentists show better results compared to the dentists with less that 10 years of experience. The method of the magnet fixing was the same for both groups, so the difference came from the personal skills for the self-curing resin treatment or surface treatment of the magnet.

Fig 10 shows the cumulative curve for keeper separation. Better results are observed for the dentists with more than 10 years of experience. The difference was statistically significant.

These results suggest that the procedure of denture with the magnetic attachment might require a lot of skill.

Summary

To conclude, the 3 most common problems we encountered over 8 year period were as follows:

- Fractures of the denture around the magnetic attachment.
- Dislodgement of the magnetic assembly from the denture base.
- Dislodgement of the keeper with coping cap.

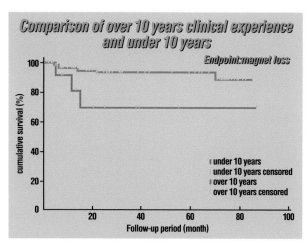

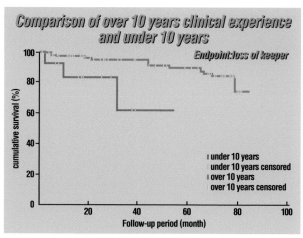

Fig 9 Comparison of performance of dentures based on the clinical experience. Endpoint : loss of magnet.

Fig 10 Comparison of performance of dentures based on the clinical experience. Endpoint : loss of keeper.

- These problems were not a result of the magnetic attachment itself but of other fundamental, procedural faults.
- For a period 8 years, all the cases showed that the retentive force of the magnetic

attachments stayed the same and did not reduce. Therefore, we can overcome these problems. Even if these problems occur, they can be easily rectified with simple repairs.

References
1. Gillings B D R, Samant A: Overdentures with magnetic attachments. Dent Clin North Am, 34: 683–709, 1990.
2. Gillings B D R: Magnetic overdentures. Aust Prosthodont J, 7: 13–21, 1993.

3. Fletcher R H, Fletcher S W, Wagner E H: Prognosis, In Clinical Epidemiology, The Essentials, 111–135, Philadelphia, Williams & Wilkins, 1996.

Chapter 12

Maintenance of Magnetically Retained Overdentures and Troubleshooting

Hiroshi Mizutani / Vygandas Rutkunas

Introduction

Overdenture treatment is far away not finished with the fabrication and insertion of it. In many instances the success or failure of overdenture treatment largely depends upon proper post insertion care, which requires number of recall visits. It is of great importance to get patient's understanding about post insertion care, oral and denture hygiene and financial implications as well. Achieving a complete cooperation of the patient is one of the main aims that in most of the cases lead to success. It is believed that success of overdenture is determined by type, design and quality of it, condition of soft and hard oral tissues at the outset of treatment and relationships of patient and dentist. Some of the studies detected significant or not differences in load transfer, denture stability and maintenance with different designs of overdenture attachments[1, 2]. Post insertion care of magnetically retained overdentures has some peculiarities.

Maintenance of Overdentures

Influence of Denture Design

One of the main advantages of tooth or implant supported overdenture over conventional complete denture is easier adaptation, higher patient satisfaction and superior masticatory efficiency, what leads to the improvement of patient's nutritional status. It restores both hard and soft tissues and provides better support for oro-facial musculature, assists in adaptation processes and is easier controlled by patient. Although the maximum bite force with fixed prosthesis is higher, maintenance of them is far more complicated and can reflect on periimplant tissue and patient satisfaction. Overdenture design possesses more freedom in artificial teeth arrangement and permits placement of them in more natural position. However, restriction of tongue space can cause discomfort, mastication and speech problems.

The importance of using a metal reinforcement in the mandibular overdenture prosthesis is still debatable as high-impact resins show low fracture rates, however, overdentures with metal base and "metal-touch" design (*Fig 1*) aid in preservation of abutments and soft tissues health due to lower rates of plaque accumulation.

Preservation of Residual Ridges and Abutments

Considering perspectives of oral health it is very important that both - remaining teeth and implants are able to control in certain extend the resorption of residual ridges. Basically the residual ridges are incapable to bear masticatory stresses. Utilizing remaining teeth or implants diminishes the loading on oral mucosa and residual ridges, and this value mainly depends on amount of support provided by abutments, opposing teeth (or prosthesis) and masticatory (para)function. According to origin of support two types of overdenture designs can be distinguished: implant

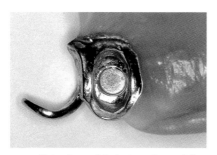

Fig 1 "Metal-touch" design of metal framework. It covers all gingival sulcus in order to lower plaque accumulation.

(tooth) supported and implant (tooth)-mucosa supported overdentures. In cleft-palate cases tooth supported overdenture is common approach. While implant-mucosa supported overdentures are common in treatment of edentulous cases.

The ability of residual ridges to tolerate masticatory stress varies largely and is influenced by general health, characteristics of masticatory forces, overdenture design and needless to say - fit of the prosthesis. Female gender is also considered as a risk factor. There are no two patients with residual ridges reacting to stress in the same way. Thus patients have to be aware of unpredictable conditions that can appear. Some studies indicate 1 mm less resorption in height of residual ridges in overdentures comparing to complete dentures in 5 years follow-up period[3].

Gaining favorable crown-root ratio after preparation diminishes occlusal loading on abutments and positively affects prognosis of them. Effective mastication, which requires tactile discrimination, relies upon feedback that is provided by periodontal mechanoreceptors, pulpal, mucosal receptors, muscle proprioreception and TMJ[4]. The limited number of implant (tooth) indicates the selection of implant (tooth)-mucosa supported overdenture and resilient attachment type. However, "stress braking" attachments are not substitute for a correctly designed and constructed denture. A poorly constructed complete denture will move around in the mouth; a poorly constructed denture with attachments will move around the roots. With very low profile and

option of "retention without bracing" magnetic attachments contribute in preservation of teeth with unfavorable periodontal status. Even temporarily preservation of hopeless teeth beneath overdenture base can facilitate use of complete dentures in the future.

Influence of Retainer Type and Design

Denture retention is defined as the resistance to vertical and torsional stresses, or the resistance of a denture to removal in a direction opposite that of its insertion[5]. Stability refers to resistance against horizontal movement and forces that tend to alter the relationship between the denture base and its supporting foundation in a horizontal or rotational direction. Investigations have found that a direct relationship exists between patient satisfaction and prosthesis retention[6] as well as stability[7]. Different retainers provide different levels of retention and stability; create different amount of stress on abutments and denture bearing area. The aim here is to adapt overdenture and retainers timely in order to prevent oral structures from excessive stress. Different retainers have different properties of fatigue and wear, therefore, maintenance is influenced by type of retainer selected. It was indicated by studies that overdentures retained by bar attachments face more complications than overdentures retained by ball attachments in the first year of service[8]. Yet mechanical attachments employing frictional forces are susceptible to wear and consequently demand more adjustment and replacing visits. As it was indicated by recent study the most common complication of all implant restoration was found to be loosening of overdenture attachment[9].

Choice of retainer depends upon several parameters: the patient's oral hygiene habits, the number and prosthodontic value of abutments, aesthetics, ability to handle denture, cost of fabrication and any additional cost should one or more abutments will be lost. Unfortunately more often than not some of remaining teeth fail to qualify as potential abutments and are subjected to extractions.

Magnetic attachments possess ability to reduce lateral forces. Thus even if candidate abutment for mechanical attachment fails to qualify as of prosthodontic value, consideration of magnetic attachment can give the positive answer. Using magnetic attachments the bracing can be easily controlled through the height and taper of root copings thus we can "administer" lateral stress to abutments according to their ability to tolerate it. So called magnetic "conic crown" can provide considerable amount of retention and bracing too, while root cap with minimal height will aid mainly in retention with minimal lateral stress transferred to abutment. Majority of retainers employ mechanical retentive elements and due to fatigue of material have to be inspected and adjusted or even replaced quite often. Initial value of retentive force of them and later changes are unpredictable, as it depends on type of mechanical retainer or even single specimen and it can decrease quite dramatically or even increase slightly (gold telescope technique). According to the results of studies precision attachments with plastic female inserts shows less wear and more consistent retentive force in comparison with precision attachments consisting of metal alloy matrix and patrix components. While magnetic attachments come up with constant retentive force in both vertical and lateral directions. That is very important as the retentive force can be easily controlled.

However magnetic attachments do have drawbacks. Earlier magnetic attachment systems were susceptible to corrosion. Modern methods of encapsulation using special types of ferromagnetic stainless steel and micro-laser welding techniques claim to overcome this problem[10]. Maximum retentive force and range of retention are small to compare with mechanical attachments.

Type of attachment influences the hygiene of abutment teeth or implants. Splinted design and considerable undercuts may contribute in accumulation of plaque and put in risk the health of periodontal or peri-implant tissues. In general the magnetic attachments are much easier to be cleaned as they have simple shape, flat surface and no undercuts. Problems still can arise as it was noticed, that with magnetically retained overdentures hygiene of abutments are less emphasized and patients could be less motivated.

Patient Satisfaction and Overdenture

The patient satisfaction is determined by multiple factors and to evaluate it is a difficult task. It is influenced by physical and by psychological factors. As the overdenture wearers are usually elderly people with a diminished ability to master new skills, retainers, requiring precise way of insertion, can form a considerable obstacle. Moreover these retainers can be even contraindicated for patients with diminished manual dexterity or with such diseases as Parkinson's. If operated improperly during overdenture insertion/removal mechanical attachments can cause excessive forces, whereas magnetically retained overdenture can be comparatively easily dislodged by sudden movement without stressing abutments and on other hand - during insertion they provide guiding forces, which assist reseating. In contrast to mechanical attachments, the bigger number of magnetic attachments is employed the easier insertion of the overdenture. That is highly appreciated by elderly patients and makes using the overdenture comfortable from the beginning.

Examination of the Overdenture

Careful periodic examination of overdenture patient is essential. The examination should involve abutment teeth, overdenture itself, oral mucosa and residual ridges, denture fitting,

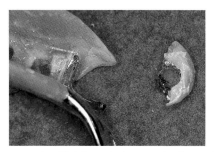

Fig 2 Aartificial tooth fracture in the region of abutment 7 years after insertion of denture.

occlusion and esthetics. After evaluation the proper adjustments have to be made and adequate preventive measures prescribed. First and most valuable information is obtained by questioning patient, paying attention to his/her complaints and remarks.

The overdenture should be inspected visually by checking for sharp edges or irregularities of the surface that can appear during processing of acrylic resin base. If found it should be carefully removed with carbide bur and polished with silicone points. Fracture or cracks of acrylic denture base tend to appear in the region of abutments where the denture base is thinnest (Fig2). As a matter of fact magnetic attachments favoring smaller dimensions than mechanical ones are easily applicable where vertical interarch distance is limited and leave more space for denture base and artificial teeth.

The visual inspection of residual ridges can provide valuable information as the sore spots on mucosa can be seen. Palpation is performed and simultaneously patient is asked about any uncomfortable feeling or severe sensation. It is recommended that patient would be aware of wearing overdenture at least 6 hours before visiting dentist as the sore spots can be diagnosed more efficiently. With time residual ridges undergo resorption and are prone to change the shape, resultant misfit can encourage residual ridge resorption further. Fast setting silicone material or disclosing paste can be used to confirm the adequacy of impression surface of overdenture

and proper extension of margins. While registering fit of denture the antagonists are prevented from any contact as the occlusal error can be transferred to record through denture shift due to presence of deflective contacts. False record of denture fitting surface can lead to damaging impression surface of denture even though it was well fitting. The lesions of mucosa in the reflections are most often caused by denture borders that are too sharp or denture flanges that are overextended. Sometimes the labial notch of the denture will be sharp or of improper shape and the frenum becomes irritated. The excessive load marks located on the slopes of residual ridges are most probably created by occlusal problems, while marks located at sulcus area are created by extra length of denture flanges. The denture border or impression surface should be adjusted with caution. Excessive shortening of flanges can reduce or eliminate the seal of the prosthesis. Also undue shortening of denture borders may decrease the denture bearing area, enhance the stresses on residual ridges and complicate interpretation of excessive pressure spots. Additional stress is placed on buccal shelf as it provides support for mandibular denture. The cause of soreness of buccal shelf should be determined. It can be caused either by improper fit of impression surface of the denture or too long buccal flange. To differentiate the cause overdenture is inserted in the mouth and level of sore spot and buccal flange is compared. Thickness of the flanges is adjusted by asking patient to smile, to open the mouth widely, to do other facial expressions and simultaneously checking the stability of denture.

The proper relieve around gingival margin of abutments teeth have to be confirmed. If pressure is detected, the excessive acrylic resin is removed. Caution should be exercised not to damage surface of magnetic assembly as scratched surface prevents magnetic assembly from close contact with keeper and can diminish retentive force of magnetic attachment. All grinded parts of denture base have to be polished as unpolished even well fitting surface may cause irritation. Also as some of the self-willed patients try to do corrections by themselves, it can be easily noticed on polished surface.

After denture bases have been checked evaluation of occlusion and articulation follows. To do this mandible is guided to IP (Intercuspal Position) by keeping finger on the mandible (chin) until first light contact. This is repeated several times and lastly patient is asked to bite down firmly. Any shift from light contact position to full intercuspation represents occlusal error. Due to mobility of mucosa the occlusion is difficult to evaluate. The occlusal error can be masked by difficult to notice denture slide on residual ridges. Therefore the occlusal relationships are easier evaluated on articulator in some cases. Occlusal corrections performed have to be coordinated with results of intra-oral examination.

Soreness on the crest of the residual ridge can develop from pressure created by heavy contacts of opposing teeth in the same region. Presence of deflective contacts may cause denture side shift and result in soreness on slopes of residual ridges or tight sensation in abutments. Also patient can complain that after insertion they feel uncomfortable with dentures but after some time the situation improves. In this case the dentist have to suspect presence of deflective occlusal contacts as later improvement of patient sensation may be related to adaptation of mucosa to stresses caused by deflective contacts and subsequent denture shift. Excessive occlusal pressure may cause generalized inflammation of denture bearing mucosa, more rare it can be the result of excessive vertical dimension of occlusion, nutritional or hormonal problems, inadequate hygiene or contact allergic reactions.

Teeth or implant supported overdenture enables the patient to exert stronger biting forces. Opposing overdenture edentulous arch (especially anterior part of maxilla) can be subjected to excessive occlusal loads and undergo resorption and fibrous replacement of residual ridge. Thus different occlusal schemes can be indicated depending upon amount of overdenture support and occlusal forces exerted by opposing arch. However when the mandibular overdenture is opposed by complete maxillary denture it is recommended to make balanced occlusion with very light anterior contacts, as the edentulous anterior maxilla is highly susceptible to occlusal stresses.

Relining, Rebasing and Remaking of the Overdentures

The occlusal load has to be evenly distributed between abutments (implant (tooth) supported overdenture) or between abutments and residual ridges (implant (tooth)-mucosa supported overdentures). As both overdentures and residual ridges inevitably undergo changes, attachments need to be replaced sometimes.

The examination of denture bases can reveal the need of relining. If occlusion is confirmed as adequate, overdenture can be relined. If the major occlusal errors are detected the rebasing or even remaking of the denture is indicated. The number of adjustments and repairs required varies largely depending on individual bone responses to occlusal load. It is also believed to be influenced by type of attachment.

Relining can be accomplished in the dental clinic or in the laboratory. Clinical procedure of relining involves removing thin layer of denture mucosal surface adding acrylic relining resin and re-fitting denture in the mouth. Thus surface of the denture is modified according to present shape of the residual ridges. Laboratory relining technique involves two steps. During clinical procedure instead of acrylic resin, the impression material or tissue conditioning material is added and the denture inserted. During laboratory step,

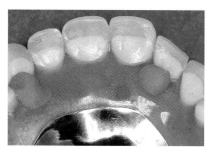

Fig 3 Spillways for draining of self-curing resin. However, it weakens the denture and can cause fracture of it.

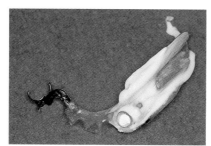

Fig 4 Magnetic denture base unfitting to the residual ridge. The thick white silicone layer shows the unfitting area.

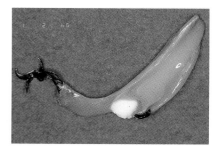

Fig 5 Magnetic denture base filled with self-curing relining resin. The magnetic assembly has to be removed before filling the relining material.

the added impression material or tissue conditioning material is substituted with acrylic resin. Both techniques have advantages and disadvantages: intra-oral technique is straightforward and costs less while laboratory one scores in safety (no chance of a chemical irritation of mucosa), color and dimension stability, and higher physical properties of acrylic resin.

Embedding of the attachment into the denture is a critical step. During curing of the resin and subsequent shrinkage of it magnetic assembly can be displaced and loose its function. Minor displacements of attachment embedded into acrylic denture are difficult to control and detect. Magnetic attachments unlike mechanical ones do not have undercuts what makes the intraoral technique relatively easier. Mechanical attachments especially bars form more obstacles as the undercuts have to be blocked. The presence of blocking material can interfere with proper placement of clips.

In order to preserve the ferromagnetic materials from high temperatures, after processing the overdenture magnetic retainer is embedded into it by self-curing resin. The spillways to drain excess of self-curing acrylic resin can be prepared in the lingual side (Fig3). It also can help to visualize the proper placement of magnetic assembly on keeper. Then through spillway hole small amount of resin is added to secure magnetic assembly to keeper. Later larger amount of resin is added to fill all remaining space around mag-

netic assembly. However, minimal amounts of self-curing resin should be employed. The smaller amount of self-curing resin cause less displacement of magnetic assembly. Performance of magnetic attachments are highly sensitive to improper orientation of them. The retention force of closed-field magnetic attachments decrease dramatically as distance between keeper and magnet increases. Thus after checking the fit of the base (Fig4) thin surface layer of denture is removed and monomer applied on surface where self-curing acrylic resin is going to be placed (Fig5). Denture facing surface of magnetic assembly is sandblasted, covered by monomer or Super Bond C&B (Sun Medicals Co. Ltd., Moriyama, Japan) and positioned properly on the root cap with keeper ensuring close contact between them (Fig6). Care is exercised to preserve the keeper-faced surface of magnetic assembly clean. The self-curing resin is placed on denture and prosthesis is reseated in the mouth carefully without applying any excessive load (Fig7). After curing of acrylic resin the overdenture is placed into the hot water to enhance polymerization. After that relief for gingival margin is made taking care not to scratch surface of magnetic assembly. It should be checked that no resin have flown between keeper and magnet (Fig8). Buccal sides and borders are finished and polished.

When the larger part of acrylic resin is going to be changed the rebasing technique is more suitable. It involves almost all laboratory steps as

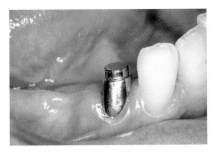

Fig 6 Magnetic assembly on the abutment with keeper. Its sandblasted surface should not be touched by hand.

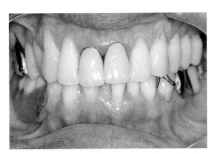

Fig 7 Magnetic denture with relining material in the mouth. Light force to keep the denture in proper position is applied while curing.

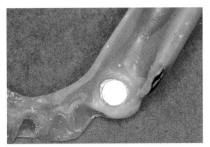

Fig 8 Magnetic denture after relining. If any resin layer is found between magnetic assembly and keeper, relining procedure must be performed again.

a making new denture and therefore is more complicated than relining. The occlusal relationships are thought to remain unchanged but during polimerization of resin they inevitably change position slightly, what makes procedure technique sensitive. In these cases remaking of the overdenture has to be considered as well.

Hygiene of Overdentures

Patients have to be educated properly to ensure hygiene of hard and soft oral tissues, and overdentures as well. The presence of plaque and calculus can be a cause of periodontitis, carious lesions, pathology of oral mucosa, halitosis and undermined esthetic appearance. Regular schedule for professional hygiene has to be set. Accumulation of plaque and inadequate oral hygiene could have effect on function of magnetic attachment. It was reported that magnet corrosion is increased in the mouth due to presence of biofilms produced by oral microflora on the surfaces and sugar levels have strong influence on production of biofiolms. The decrease in mass of the Nd-Fe-B magnets was 28-fold greater in the presence of sucrose than with its absence. Plaque control consists of cleaning abutments, oral mucosa and overdentures. Single tooth brush specially designed for root cap is used for prevention of abutments (Fig 9, 10). If the periodontal pocked is deep (more than 4 mm) the use of interdental brush is advised (Fig 11). Ordinary soft toothbrush is used for cleaning oral mucosa

and tongue (Fig 12). Cleaning of the overdentures has to be done after every meal. Patients have to be discouraged from using toothpastes containing abrasives. Special denture cleaning agents can be also used as they don't cause corrosion of magnets. During night dentures are removed from the mouth and placed in container with water (Fig 13). Prescribing plaque staining tablets helps patient to evaluate efficiency of hygiene. Minimum twice a year professional hygiene of the abutments is performed. Applications of fluoride gel were proved as highly efficient preventive measure against caries. Overdenture itself can be used as a tray for fluoride gel application.

Troubleshooting

Some of the common problems with magnetically retained overdentures and solutions for them follow:

• Magnetic attachments for patient with pacemaker.

Magnetic attachment are located remotely from pacemaker. Even if the magnetic denture itself is placed in the left pocket of the shirt- the closest proximity do not have any ill effects on the work of pacemaker. However, it is recommended to select non-magnetic retainer for these patients.

• Biologic effects of magnetic field.

The magnetic field leakage of currently available closed-field magnetic attachment systems is around 0.004 T, while 0.02 T is considered as a safety standard. Currently available evidence sug-

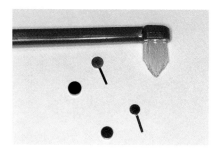

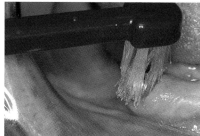

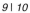

Fig 9 Single tooth brush designed for cleaning of root cap.
Fig 10 Single tooth brush used in the mouth in order to maintain the hygiene of abutment.

9 | 10

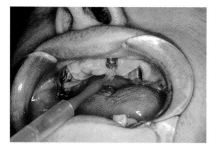

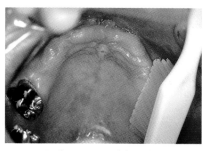

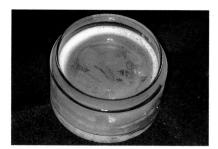

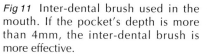

Fig 11 Inter-dental brush used in the mouth. If the pocket's depth is more than 4mm, the inter-dental brush is more effective.

Fig 12 Ordinary toothbrush used to clean soft tissues.

Fig 13 Magnetic denture dipped in denture cleaner. Ordinary denture cleaner sold on the market can be used without any fear of corrosion.

gests that the conceivable risks of harmful biological effects of magnetic attachments are negligible. In addition, the magnetic field is always constant and its not so harmfull as alternating one like in some electric equipments: microwave oven, electric shaver, TV etc.,

• Fracture of the abutment resin tooth.

Overdentures get support from abutments and denture base, and their compression rates are very different from each other. Thus all overdentures tend to fracture in the region of abutments. Solutions: selection of magnetic attachment with lower profile or placement of metal artificial tooth.

• Restricted vertical space

Solutions: preparation of deeper recess in occlusal surface of root, magnetic attachments with low profile, metal base reinforcement, placement of metal artificial tooth.

• Unparallel abutments

The magnetic attachments don't call for precise alignment. Solution: keepers are set unparallel with maximum deviation of 10∞ to occlusal plane.

• Planned MRI examination

Before taking MRI (Magnetic Resonance Imaging), the magnetic denture (including the magnetic assembly) should be removed; otherwise the image is notedly damaged. While the presence of keeper (ferromagnetic materials) in the mouth during MRI examination can cause a minor degradation of image (Fig 14), especially when structures in proximity of keeper are investigated, e.g. TMJ disk. Area of MRI affected by keeper, is said to be of the golf-ball size. Thus any main organs or tissues except TMJ disks are safely taken if the denture is removed. Solutions: however, a screw-retained keeper is available in case of MRI of TMJ disks (Fig 15, 16). Record is made in the patient file that he/she has magnetic attachment.

• Candidate root for abutment is below gingival margin

Solutions: the same magnetic attractive force can be applied to perform root extrusion. However, the consequent change of crown/root ratio have to be considered.

• Dislodged magnetic assembly

The design of magnetic assembly varies among makers and different models. Some of magnetic assemblies incorporate special retentive

104

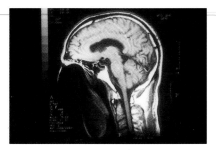

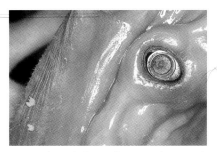

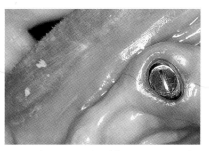

Fig 14 MRI image with keeper. Any organs or tissues except these in proximity of keeper (e.g. TMJ disks) are safely taken if the denture is removed.

Fig 15 Threaded metal cap in the mouth with keeper removed.

Fig 16 Screw-retained keeper set in the root cap.

elements - undercuts, wings etc. If the magnetic assembly without retentive elements is dislodged from acrylic base and the reason is identified as bad adhesion of assembly to the base, sandblasting and use of adhesive should solve the problem. Otherwise assemblies with special retentive elements can be employed.

• Dislodgement of keeper

Cemented keepers can be cemented again followed by relocation of magnetic assembly in denture base. Root caps if decemented have to be remade after creating more retentive form of preparation.

• Corrosion of the keeper

Also recent magnetic attachments claim to be protected from corrosion, cast bonded keepers, because of the casting imperfections and resultant crevice formed between keeper and casting, can exhibit crevice corrosion. Solution: keeper has to be changed.

• Diminished retention of overdenture.

Solutions: re-embed the magnetic assembly or relining the overdenture.

References

1. Tokuhisa M, Matsushita Y, Koyano K: In vitro study of a mandibular implant overdenture retained with ball, magnet, or bar attachments: comparison of load transfer and denture stability. Int J Prosthodont, 16(2): 128−314, 2003.

2. Duyck J, Van Oosterwyck H, Vander Sloten J, De Cooman M, Puers R, Naert I: In vivo forces on oral implants supporting a mandibular overdenture: the influence of attachment system. Clin Oral Investig, 3(4): 201−207, 1999.

3. Kordatzis K, Wright P S, Meijer H J: Posterior mandibular residual ridge resorption in patients with conventional dentures and implant overdentures. Int J Oral Maxillofac Implants, 18(3): 447−452, 2003.

4. Jacobs R, van Steenberghe D: Role of periodontal ligament receptors in the tactile function of teeth: a review. J Periodontal Res, 29(3): 153−167, 1994.

5. The Academy of Prosthodontics. Glossary of Prosthodontic Terms. J Prostet Dent, 71: 50−107, 1994.

6. Naert I, Quirynen M, Theuniers G, van Steenberghe D: Prosthetic aspects of osseointegrated fixtures supporting overdentures. A 4-year report. J Prosthet Dent, 65(5): 671−680, 1991.

7. Feine J S, de Grandmont P, Boudrias P, Brien N, LaMarche C, Tache R, Lund J P: Within-subject comparisons of implant-supported mandibular prostheses: choice of prosthesis. J Dent Res, 73(5): 1105−1111, 1994.

8. Gotfredsen K, Holm B: Implant-supported mandibular overdentures retained with ball or bar attachments: a randomized prospective 5-year study. Int J Prosthodont, 13(2): 125−130, 2000.

9. Goodacre CJ, Bernal G, Rungcharassaeng K, Kan JY. Clinical complications with implants and implant prostheses. J Prosthet Dent, 90(2): 121−32, 2003.

10. Walmsley A D, Frame J W: Implant supported overdentures−the Birmingham experience. J Dent, 25: Suppl 1, 43−47, 1997.

Part 3

Clinical Cases

Clinical cases

In this section, 25 cases of conventional removable dentures and 2 cases of implant retained dentures using magnetic attachments are presented.

Cases of canventional removable denture

The cases were classified according to number of magnetic attachment applied.

Number of MA	Jaws	Cases
1	Upper	1, 3, 4, 7, 10, 15, 25
	Lower	2, 5, 6, 13, 14, 16
2	Upper	11, 13
	Lower	4, 8, 9, 19, 22, 23
3	Upper	20, 21
	Lower	12, 17
4	Upper	13, 24
	Lower	/

In 9 cases, only magnetic attachment is used as the retainer of the denture, while in the rest, magnetic attachment is used together with other conventional retainers such as clasp (C), telescope crown (T) or root surface attachment (A).

Case	Retainer	Case	Retainer	Case	Retainer	Case	Retainer
1	M	8	M	15	+A	23	M
2	+C	9	M	16	+T	24	+C
3	+T	10	+C	17	M	25	+C
4U	+T	11	M	18	M		
L	+T	12	M	19	+C		
5	+T	13U	+C	20	M		
6	+C	13L	+C	21	+C		
7	+C	14	+C	22	+C		

Cases of implant retained denture

Two magnetic attchments are used to the implant in each case.

Case 1
Replacement of a Damaged Root Surface Attchment—1

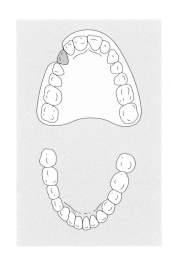

Patient: 60 years old, female

Chief complaint: Instability of the upper denture

Remaining teeth: 13, 31−37, 41−47

Location of magnetic attachments: 13

Reasons for use of magnetic attachments: Replacement of a damaged stud attachment

Initial Situation

The patient came with the complaint that the upper denture, which was made about one year ago, became loose. It was found on the examination that the root surface attachment fixed to the only remaining tooth 13(*Fig1*) was broken and lost its retentive function. Special findings were not obtained except for a slight mobility of the abutment root. There was no problem with the fitting of the denture. The patient has full teeth in the lower jaw.

Treatment Plan and Procedures

The damaged attachment was to be removed and replaced with a new retentive appliance. Magnetic attachment Magfit EX 600 was applied on account of the protection of the moving abutment. Since the vertical space between the upper and lower jaws was little, the root surface was prepared below the level of gingival margin. As the result, the surface was inclined because the root was located buccally. It is important for the proper retentive force of magnetic attachments that the keeper should be set parallel to the occlusal plane. In this case, however, if this requirement was indicated, sufficient room for the magnet could not be obtained. Then, the keeper had to be set in a leaning position (*Fig2*). In addition, in order to make the room enough for the magnet, the root cap was prepared so that the keeper was set lower than the surface of the cap (*Fig3,4*).

In spite of these measures, inside corner of the root cap projected in the mouth (*Fig5*), and the denture was expected to become thin in this part when the magnet was fixed. But, the magnet was fixed to the denture by usual way and the repair of the denture was finished (*Fig6*). The denture regained retention and the patient was satisfied.

Outcome of Treatment

After about one and a half years, the denture was cracked at inside of the abutment 13 and artificial canine came off (*Fig7*). Damaged part of the denture was repaired, but the same part was damaged repeatedly since then. So, it was reinforced by a metal plate (*Fig8*).

At the present of about five and a half years since the denture was set, it works well without any troubles (*Fig9, 10*). During the period, maintenance was performed every six months.

Magnetic attachments were frequently used at canines. In the case of buccally dislocated canines, the prepared surface of the roots is apt to be inclined as shown in this case. If the keeper is fixed parallel to the occlusal plane, buccal side of the root cap has to be made tall. In such the shape, esthetical problem takes place such as artificial teeth of the overdenture project buccally or become thin and sometimes the metal of the root cap can be seen through the artificial teeth. In this case, as the vertical space was little, magnetic attachment was

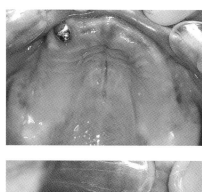

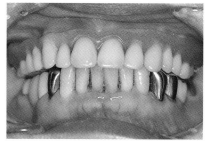

Fig 1 Stud attachment in the mouth before damaged.
Fig 2 The root cap with the keeper was fixed to the abutment 13

1 | 2

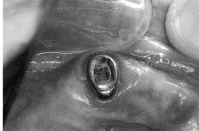

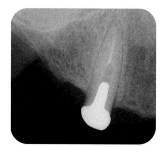

Fig 3 The keeper was set below the surface of the cap.
Fig 4 The abutment was in good condition on the X-ray photo.

3 | 4

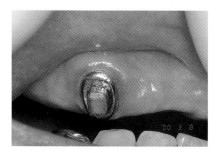

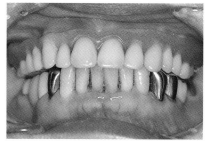

Fig 5 Inside corner of the magnet projected and approached the lower teeth.
Fig 6 The denture with the magnet in the mouth.

5 | 6

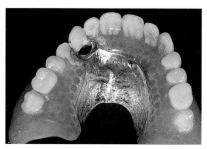

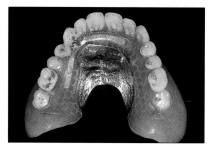

Fig 7 The denture damaged after about one and a half years.
Fig 8 The denture reinforced with a metal plate.

7 | 8

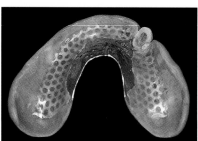

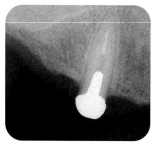

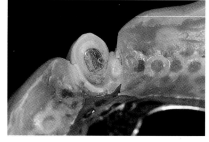

Fig 9 Inner surface of the denture after five and a half years.

Fig 10 The abutment was kept well after five and a half years.

Fig 11 Partial attrition was seen on the attractive surface of the magnet.

used obliquely, but still the denture became thin at the part. Magfit EX 600 was used here, the height of which is 2.8mm. At the present, much lower magnetic attachments are in the market and these problems may hardly take place.

In addition, the overdenture with one abutment is prone to move around the abutment, and the denture and the abutment tooth may be damaged by overload. Partial attrition is often seen on the attractive surfaces of the magnet and the keeper (*Fig 11*). Regular maintenance is particularly important.

(Seiichiro Someya)

Case 2
Replacement of a Damaged Root Surface Attchment—2

Patient: 73 years old, female

Chief complaint: Food impaction around 43 tooth

Remaining teeth: 31, 32, 41–43, 48

Location of magnetic attachments: 43

Reason for use of magnetic attachments: No crown of 43, high requirements for hygiene

Initial Situation

The patient referred to clinic with complaints of food impaction beneath the lower denture base. Also she complained of bleeding gums and unsatisfactory stability of the denture. Upper arch was completely edentulous (*Fig 1a*), while 31, 32, 41, 42 were splinted with gold onlays from lingual side and root of 43 tooth had Dalla Bona spherical attachment (*Fig 1b*). The gingival tissues around attachment were inflammatory, the root was affected by secondary caries which resulted in bad fit of attachment and accumulation of plaque (*Fig 1c*).

Treatment Planning and Procedures

The remaining teeth were scaled and the carious tissues from 43 tooth were removed. To increase stability of the denture and ease of hygiene of 43 tooth, the root cap with bracing properties with magnetic attachment treatment was selected. Cast-bonded Hicorex 3513 (Hitachi Metals, Japan) keeper was attached to root cap cast from Ag-Pd-Au alloy. The height and taper of root cap enable to provide more retention to lower partial overdenture (*Fig 2*). After root cap cementation and taking impressions the new upper complete denture and lower partial overdenture were made (*Fig 3a*). Upper complete denture involved full palatal coverage by metal major connector in order to distribute more evenly occlusal loads and to diminish thickness of prosthesis in palatal area (*Fig 3b*). The lower partial overdenture construction involved lingual major connector, ring clasp on 48 tooth and wire clasp on 32 for balanced retention and minimized loading of lower 32 tooth during displacement of overdenture (*Fig 3c*). The meticulous hygiene of 43 tooth was emphasized and schedule for follow-up appointments was set.

Fig 1a–c Dental condition upon presentation

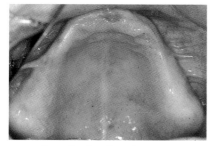

Fig 1a Completely edentulous upper.

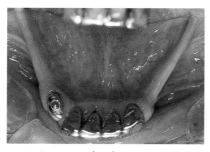

Fig 1b Lower occlusal view. 31, 32, 41, 42 were splinted with gold onlays.

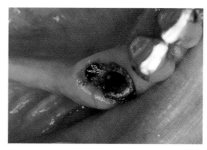

Fig 1c A metal cap with Dalla Bona spherical attachment were removed and secondary caries in the 43 root was observed.

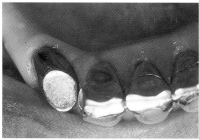

Fig 2 A keeper bonded root cap with 3mm height was set in the mouth.

Fig 3a–c New upper and lower dentures.

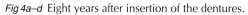

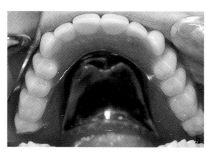

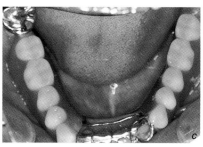

Fig 3a Occlusal view of upper and lower dentures. The posterior border of the upper denture was covered with resin in order to be able to seal the space.

Fig 3b A upper complete denture set in the mouth.

Fig 3c A lower partial overdenture set in the mouth.

Fig 4a–d Eight years after insertion of the dentures.

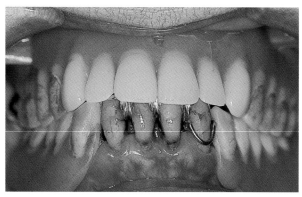

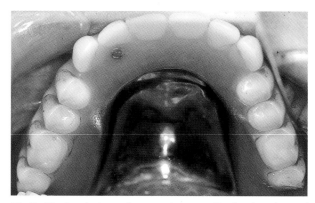

Fig 4a Frontal view of the mouth with the dentures. Buccal surface of the posterior teeth were all stained.

Fig 4b Occlusal view of upper denture. Occlusal surface of the posterior teeth were evenly worn out.

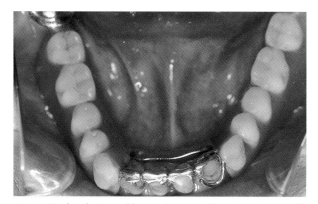

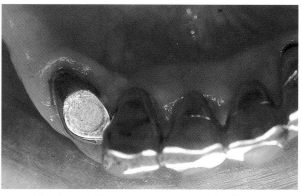

Fig 4c Occlusal view of lower denture. The ring clasp on 48 tooth and wire clasp on 32 tooth were fit well respectively.

Fig 4d Metal cap with the keeper on 43 tooth. There were no signs of inflammation and corrosion.

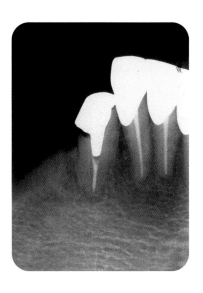

Fig5 X-ray photo of lower 43 after 8 years after insertion of the dentures. Secondary caries was observed in the distal side, but conservative treatment was recommended considering her age.

Outcome of Treatment

The patient was recalled every 3 months. During period of 8 years the upper and lower dentures were relined only once. After 8 years of follow-up periods, the enamel of lower incisors underwent discoloration (*Fig4a*). Since there were no detected secondary caries around onlay splint and the patient has no complaints about esthetics, they were continued for follow up. The retention and stability of upper and lower dentures were in good condition and mastication reported by patient as efficient (*Fig4a,b*). The keeper surface was scratched slightly without any significant loss of retention and the gingival tissues around root cap were with minor inflammation (*Fig3d*). Even though the radiograph of 43 tooth revealed secondary caries near root cap (*Fig5*), considering patient's age and request for conservative treatment option it is recommended to restore the root with composite resin.

(Hiroshi Mizutani／Vygandas Rutkunas)

Case 3
Replacement of a Damaged Telescope Crown—1

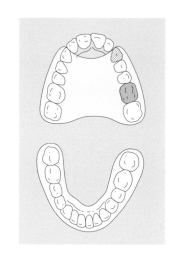

Patient: 61 years old, female

Chief complaint: Shedding of inner crown and instability of upper telescope crown retained denture

Remaining teeth: 12, 11, 21-23, 26, 31, 42, 44

Locations of magnetic attachments: 26

Reasons for use of magnetic attachments: Recovery of denture retention after break of telescope crown

Initial Situation

The patient had upper partial denture retained by cone telescope crowns at the teeth 23, 26 and lower complete overdenture (*Fig 1, 2*). Originally, 8 years ago, the upper denture was retained by telescope crowns at 14, 23 and 26 but one year ago 14 was extracted according to the root fracture. Inner crown and metal coping of 26 were lost and the root surface was exposed in the mouth with caries (*Fig 3*). The caries was found above the level of alveolar bone crest and any invasion was not observed around the furcation and the apex of the roots. There was no problem in the periodontal tissue with pocket depth of about 2mm (*Fig 4*). The upper denture almost lost its retention for lack of telescope crown of 26.

Treatment Planning and Procedure

Repair of the telescope crown was planned first but it was found difficult to make inner crown with metal coping so as to fit well to the existed outer crown, and it was proper to make new denture. The remaining root of 26 was decided to be available for abutment because the caries was limited superficially and the periodontal condition was fairy well. It was temporarily decided that the denture was repaired by using magnetic attachment in the root of 26. Magfit EX600 was suitable in size for setting its magnetic assembly into the outer telescope crown. Attractive surface of the keeper was adjusted in making wax pattern of the root coping so as to be parallel to the occlusal plane (*Fig 5, 6*). The coping with keeper was fixed to the abutment with adhesive cement (*Fig 7*) and magnetic assembly was set into the outer crown of the denture with autopolymerizing resin as usual technique (*Fig 8*). The denture was retained well and recovered in function (*Fig 9*). The patient regained good chewing function and was satisfied with this repairs.

Outcome of Treatment

The patient was recalled regularly after the treatment. Good condition as in the repairs was observed at the recall after four years (*Fig 10*).

(Motonobu Miyao)

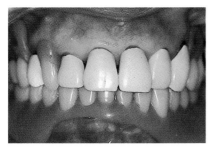

Fig 1 Initial situation of the upper and lower dentures in the mouth.
Fig 2 The upper and lower dentures.

1 | 2

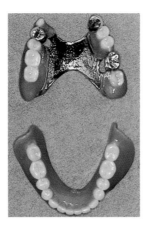

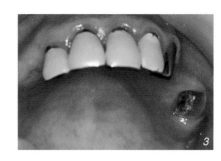

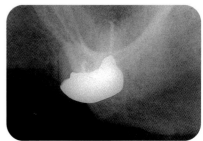

Fig 3 The inner crown of abutment tooth 26 was shed.
Fig 4 Condition of the root surface of the tooth 26.

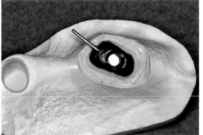

5 | 6

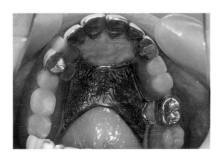

Fig 5 Wax-up of the coping with a keeper of the tooth 26.
Fig 6 Adjustment of the keeper using a mandrel with a magnet.

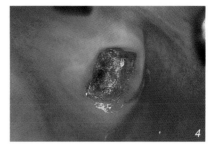

7 | 8

Fig 7 The coping with the keeper set to the abutment tooth 26.
Fig 8 The magnetic assembly fixed to the denture.

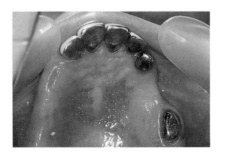

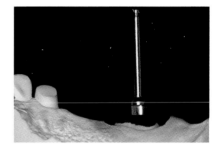

9 | 10

Fig 9 The repaired denture set in the mouth.
Fig 10 X-ray photo of the abutment after 4 years.

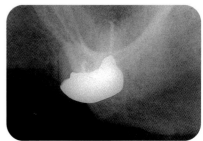

Case 4
Replacement of a Damaged Telescope Crown—2

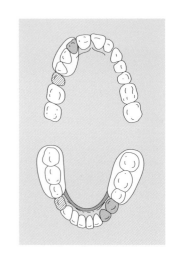

Patient: 78 years old, female

Chief complaint: Instability of the lower denture

Remaining teeth: 17, 16, 12, 11, 21–23, 25–27, 31–34, 41–44, 48

Location of magnetic attachments: 12, 33, 34

Reasons for use of magnetic attachments: Repair of the dentures with telescope crowns

Initial Situation

The patient complained of instability of the lower denture which she had used with satisfaction for about eleven years. The upper and lower dentures were retained with cone telescope crowns. It was found on the examination that the inner telescope crown of the abutment tooth 33 was lost and only the root remained (*Fig 1*). It was kept in good condition though some caries was partially seen on the surface (*Fig 2*).

Treatment Plan and Procedures

It was very difficult to remake the inner crown according to the outer crown. Then, the denture was decided to be repaired by using magnetic attachment.

The root cap with the keeper was made as usual. Taking account of easiness of brushing and expecting some bracing effect for the denture, the cap was designed high from the gingiva (*Fig 3, 4*). The magnet Magfit 600 was fixed in the outer crown with autopolymerizing resin so as to fit to the keeper (*Fig 5*). The denture became stable and regained good function.

About one and a half years later, the abutment 34 was broken (*Fig 6*). The reason of this was thought that the overload exerted on the abutment according to unbalanced occlusal stress possibly caused by damage of abutment 33. The repair was performed using same magnetic attachment Magfit 600 as used before (*Fig 7*).

After about one year, the inner crown of the abutment 12 was shed and was repaired with magnetic attachment Hicorex 3013 by the same way as before. The dentures were restored and no problem was observed in morphology and function (*Fig 8*).

Outcome of Treatment

The patient appeared after one and a half years' absence. She had been ill in bed.

Unevenness was slightly observed in the fitness of the dentures but the patient was satisfied with them. After that, she was hospitalized and could not come again.

The telescope crown system is an excellent technique for the retention of dentures but it has a disadvantage that the inner crown is apt to come off or be broken in its long use. Besides it is indeed difficult to repair this as it was. But, the denture can be restored by using magnetic attachments and its function is regained easily.

(Seiichiro Someya)

Fig 1 The residual root of the abutment 33 where the inner telescope crown had been indicated.
Fig 2 Good condition was seen on the X-ray photo of the root 33.

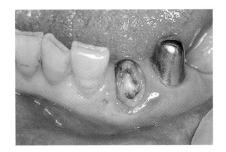
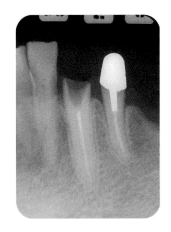

1 | 2

Fig 3 Tall root cap with the keeper was designed. The magnet is on the keeper.
Fig 4 X-ray photo of the root cap fixed to the root 33.

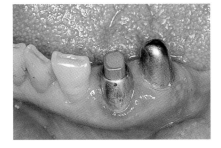
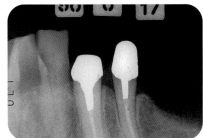

3 | 4

Fig 5 The magnet was fixed in the outer crown.
Fig 6 The abutment 34 was damaged.

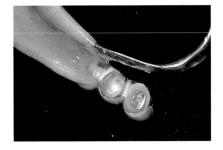
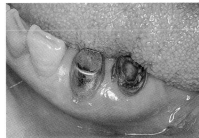

5 | 6

Fig 7a, b X-ray photo of the abutment root 34 before(a) and after(b) recovery with the magnetic attachment.

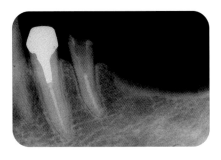
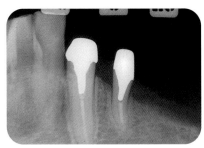

a | b

Fig 8 The dentures in the mouth after repair of the abutment 12.

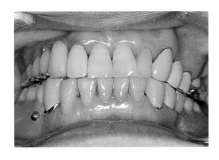

Case 5
Replacement of a Damaged Telescope Crown—3

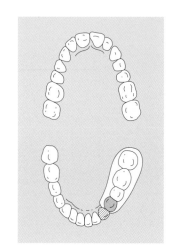

Patient: 50 years old, female

Chief complaint: Masticatory disorder

Remaining teeth: 11–15, 17, 21–27, 31–34, 41–45, 47

Location of magnetic attachments: 34

Reasons for use of magnetic attachments: Reinforcing denture retention

Initial Situation

This lady came from the department of endodontics in the university clinic of our dental school. Chief complaint was masticatory disorder caused by the loss of bilateral posterior occlusal support in lower jaw. She treated almost of all her teeth due to generalized caries for long years. Right quadrant was restored by the fixed partial denture.

Since, left side teeth loss was a distal extension one, the use of removable partial denture with unilateral design was highly indicated. The unilateral telescope distal extension RPD was first designed with the vital abutments both on 33 and 34. After the initial preparation with removal of the old full coverage restoration to the temporary one on 34, it was involved undermining cervical caries on the distal surface of the abutment.

X-ray photo revealed the poor tooth structure of the abutment 34. The estimated distal abutment 34 fractured in the course of the preprosthetic treatment, and it was highly indicated to utilize the root retainer with a mechanical or magnetic attachment, since we had many experiences of the root fracture of the telescope retainers on the devitalized abutment even with metal dowel core. The abutment had nevertheless endodontically treated. (Fig 1–3)

Treatment Plan and Procedures

Since, she had no experience to wear lower denture for years, unilateral distal extension RPD was indicated with telescope retainer on 33 and root retainer based on the magnetic attachment on 34 with distal extension saddle. Periodontal condition around the abutment was good, the abutment 33 was prepared accepting a primary crown of the telescope and 34 was prepared for root cap retainer (Fig 4).

Cp-titanium was applied to make a primary and secondary crown of the telescope retainer and associated removable part of the prosthesis. The root cap retainer incorporating a magnetic keeper of the Magfit EX 600 was first made in a usual manner.

The outline of the distal extension saddle was decided to cover the necessary tissue support from the residual ridge on the left mandible .

The complete small unilateral distal extension denture was first fabricated without the magnetic attachment on 34 only by the frictional retention by the telescope retainer on 33. After incorporation of the denture with slight sinking of the saddle, the magnetic attachment was fixed by self curing resin into place (Fig 5). The galvanic action was observed on the 33 in occlusion with the antagonistic full coverage restoration, the reacted surface was reduced for safety. She was accustomed to the restoration with good esthetic result (Fig 6–8).

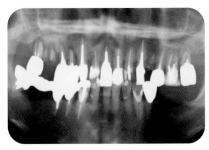

Fig 1 Panoramic X-ray photo indicated expanded caries susceptibility of this lady with many treatment histories.

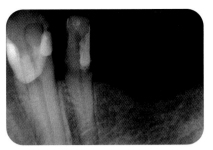

Fig 2 X-ray photo revealed the distal defect after removal of the existing full coverage crown on 34.

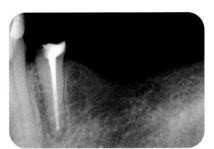

Fig 3 Endodontic treatment was proceeded for the final restorative treatment.

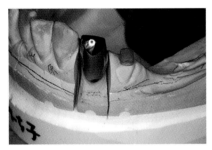

Fig 4 Combined telescope and magnetic attachment retained unilateral distal extension RPD was made.

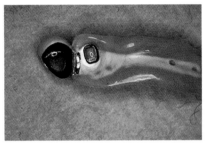

Fig 5 Cp-titanium was utilized to make the primary and secondary telescopes and associated denture frameworks. Magfit EX 600 was applied to the inner housing made of Cp-titanium with Super-Bond C & B.

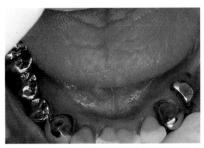

Fig 6 Lower jaw accepting the unilateral distal extension RPD with telescope primary crown on 33 and metal coping with keeper on 34.

Fig 7 The denture in situ with rigid recovery for the continuous artificial occlusion.
Fig 8 Esthetic recovery in the lower left quadrant with the RPD in situ.

7 | 8

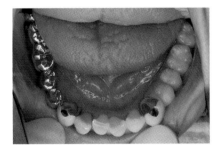

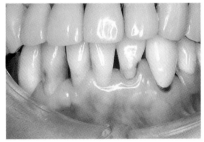

Outcome of Treatment

She declared the looseness of the denture for the first time. The secondary telescope crown was adjusted to give more retention for her request. She was able to eat almost any food with this prosthesis with natural expression by laughing and conversation.

Clinical supporting therapy for this patient has executed every 4 months per year. She wore this prosthesis one and a half year from the initial fabrication.

(Yoshimasa Igarashi)

Case 6
Replacement of a Damaged Crown

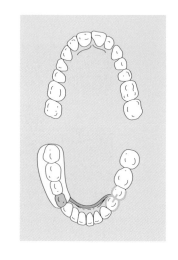

Patient: 50 years old, female

Chief complaint: Detachment of lower cantilever bridge

Remaining teeth: 11–17, 21–27, 31–35, 37, 41–45

Location of magnetic attachments: 44

Reasons for use of magnetic attachments: Esthetically good appealing and restricted interocclusal space.

Initial Situation

The patient complained of detachment of 44, 45 cantilever bridge (*Fig 1a–c*). In the past radiograph of the bridge (*Fig 2*), the unfavorable anatomy of 44, 45 roots, insufficient length of posts and caries of 45 tooth can be seen. Distal extension bridge and increased occlusal load from natural antagonists could be considered as reasons of bridge failure as well.

Treatment Planning and Procedures

The 45 tooth was indeed damaged by caries and was extracted. The restoration of 44 tooth by crown and subsequent fabrication of removable partial denture was contraindicated, because 44 tooth could not provide adequate support and was exposed to be fractured. The partial overdenture construction was indicated. Due to limitation of vertical space the application of magnetic attachment was selected. The 44 root was pre-

pared for root cap with creating ferrule effect in order to strengthen abutment (*Fig 3*). The root cap with cast bonded keeper Hicorex Super J 4015 was made and cemented with adhesive resin Super–Bond C&B (*Fig 4*). Note the limitation of vertical space available. The new lower partial overdenture was fabricated. The bracing of the denture was not enough only with this one abutment and the indirect retainer by double Akers clasps were designed on 34, 35 teeth (*Fig 5*). As small mechanical retention provided by the indirect retainer and root cap was enough, it was postponed to embed the magnetic assembly in the denture. After having conditioned the oral tissue for 3 months, the magnetic assembly was embedded in the denture by brush-up technique with auto polymerizing resin (*Fig 6*). The oral hygiene and importance of maintenance was emphasized. The patient was satisfied with denture retention and reported comfortable mastication.

Fig 1a–c Dental condition upon presentation. Patient claimed the detachment of the distal extension bridge.

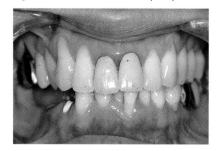

Fig 1a Frontal view of the mouth.

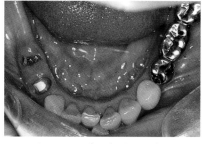

Fig 1b Lower occlusal view. The caries reached deeply below the gingival level on the 45 tooth.

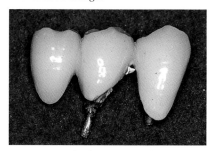

Fig 1c Detached extension bridge (44, 45).

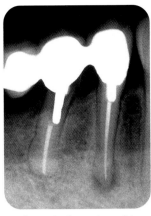

Fig2 X-ray photo before detaching. Second caries was observed on the 45 tooth. The post length was extremely short compared to the root length of the 44 tooth.

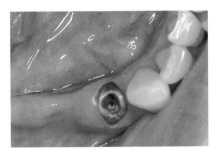

Fig3 Prepared 44 tooth for the magnetic attachment.

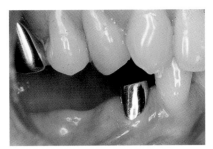

Fig4 A metal cap with the keeper cemented on the 44 abutment tooth. Interocclusal spade was very limited.

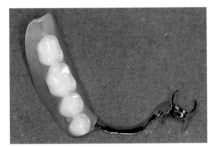

Fig5 A new fabricated lower denture.

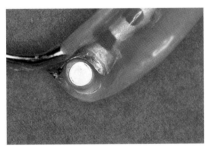

Fig6 The inner surface of the denture 3 months after setting. The magnetic assembly had not been cemented during this period.

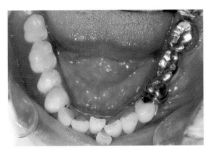

Fig7 The Denture set in the mouth 3 years after first insertion. It was firstly relined because its displacement was noticeable by finger pressure.

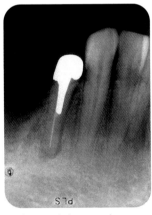

Fig8 X-ray photo of the 44 abutment tooth 3 years after the denture setting. No changes in bone level was observed compared to the 'before treatment stage'.

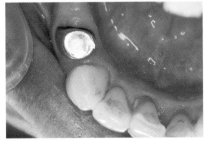

Fig9 Occlusal surface of the keeper 5 years after the denture setting.

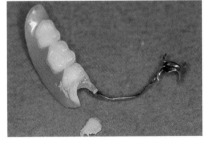

Fig10 The lower denture 7 years after setting. The artificial tooth was broken.

Outcome of Treatment

Three years after the denture setting, displacement of lower partial overdenture was detectable and the denture was relined intraorally (Fig7). The radiograph of 44 abutment didn't indicate any changes in bone level or periodontal disease (Fig8). Five years after the denture setting, the magnetic attachment had no clinically significant loss of retention, though minor scratches could be seen on surface of keeper (Fig9). Seven years after the denture setting, the patient addressed the clinic with complaint of broken artificial

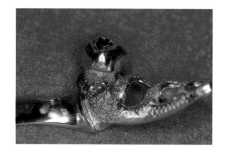

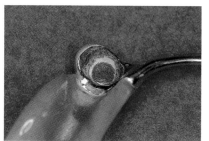

Fig 11 A new cast crown laser welded to the lower pre-existing metal framework. In order to reinforce the fracture resistance, the metal made appliance was utilized.
Fig 12 A new magnetic assembly cemented in the metal crown.

11 | 12

13 | 14

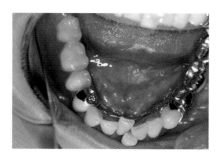

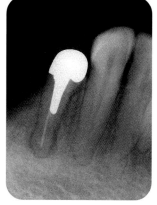

Fig 13 The lower denture with new metal tooth on the 44 tooth set in the mouth.
Fig 14 X-ray photo of the lower 44 tooth 10 years after the initial treatment. No signs of periodontal diseases were observed.

tooth (*Fig 10*). The increased occlusal loads and insufficient thickness of acrylic resin due to space limitation were the main reason of failure. To increase resistance of 44 artificial tooth, an acrylic faced metal cast crown enable to contain the magnetic assembly were employed. Initially the impression of lower dental arch was taken with this lower denture. Then, acrylic denture base with artificial teeth were removed from the framework and cast crown was fabricated and laser welded to the framework (*Fig 11*). The acrylic denture base with artificial teeth and acrylic facing cast crown were processed on the framework and Hicorex Hyperslim 4013 magnetic assembly embedded by auto polymerizing acrylic resin (*Fig 12*). The partial overdenture was seated in the mouth and is in use without any problems (*Fig 13*). Four times a year the patient is scheduled for scaling and re-checking fit of partial overdenture. Minimal bone loss and good marginal fit could be seen in the radiograph done 10 years after root cap placement (*Fig 14*).

(Hiroshi Mizutani／Vygandas Rutkunas)

Case 7
Improvement of Poor Retention of Upper Denture

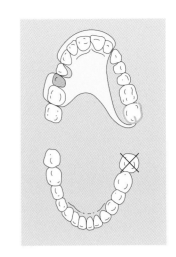

Patient: 64 years old, male

Chief complaint: Shedding of inlay and poor retention of upper denture

Remaining teeth: 17, 15, 14, 22, 23, 25–27, 31–36, 41–47

Locations of magnetic attachments: 15

Reasons for use of magnetic attachments:

Improvement of denture retention

Initial Situation

The patient came with complaint of shedding of inlay from the tooth and poor retention of upper partial denture. It is found that the poor denture retention was caused by disabled retentive function of abutment tooth 15 due to shedding of the inlay.

Inspection and X-ray examination of the abutment tooth showed the necessity of root treatment and improvement of its CR ratio, because the tooth was rather mobile with considerable periodontal involvement (*Fig 1*).

The denture which was made about two years ago was retained by clasps at 17 and 27 and by magnetic attachment Hicorex MD500 at 22 (*Fig 2, 3*).

Treatment Planning and Procedures

The patient was accustomed to use this denture and did not wish to have new denture though the clasp at 27 was also broken. Mobility of the denture was not observed horizontally. Then, the denture was decided to be repaired.

The tooth 15 was treated as usual (*Fig 4*). For the recovery of denture retention and improvement of CR ratio of the tooth 15, application of magnetic attachment was recommended and the oval type of the keeper was selected according to the outline of the root surface. The keeper was fixed to the root by DC-Core dual cure resin cement after treatment by Super-bond C&B (*Fig 5*). The magnetic assembly Magfit EX600W was fixed to the denture with autpolymerizing resin as usual way (*Fig 6, 7*). By using magnetic attachment, retention of the upper denture was improved and the patient was satisfied.

Outcome of Treatment

About one year has past since the repairs. The prognosis is fairy well (*Fig 8*). Periodontal condition on the X-ray photo and mobility of the tooth 15 was improved compared with the initial situation (*Fig 9*).

The magnetic atttachment at 22 had been in good function for three years but the assembly came off few months ago. As any damage was not observed, it was reset in the denture. Severe wear or corrosion was not observed on the attractive surfaces of both magnetic attachments (*Fig 8, 10*) and the denture functions well at present (*Fig 11, 12*).

(Shinsuke Sadamori)

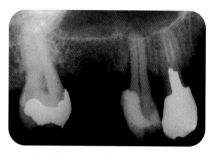
Fig 1   Initial X-ray photo of the tooth 15.

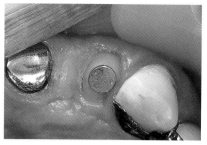
Fig 2   The keeper fixed to the tooth 22.

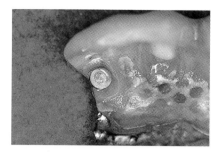
Fig 3   The magnetic assembly fixed to the denture.

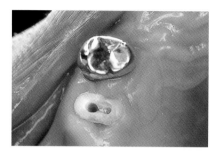

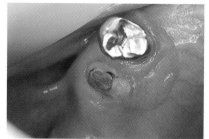

4 | 5

Fig 4   The tooth 15 was prepared for the magnetic attachment application.
Fig 5   The keeper was fixed to the root of the tooth 15.

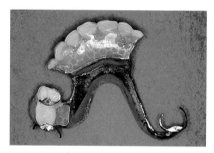

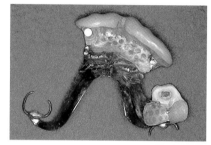

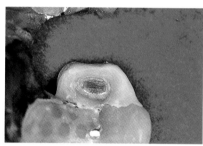

Fig 6a, d   The upper denture repaired by using magnetic attachment. a: Artificial tooth was fixed to the region of the tooth 15.   b: The magnetic assembly was set in the denture.

a | b

Fig 7   The magnetic assembly at the region of 15 of the denture.

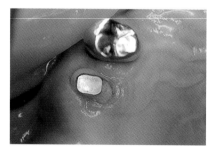

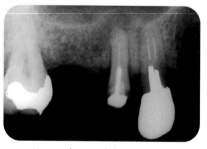

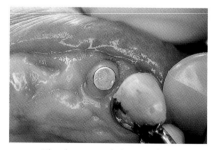

Fig 8   The keeper of the tooth 15 after about one year.

Fig 9   X-ray photo of the tooth root 15 after about one year.

Fig 10   The keeper of the tooth 22 after four years.

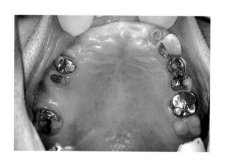

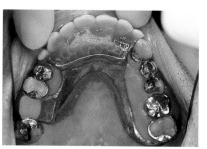

11 | 12

Fig 11   Remaining teeth of the upper jaw.
Fig 12   The upper denture in the mouth.

Case 8
Improvement of Poor Retention of Lower Denture—1

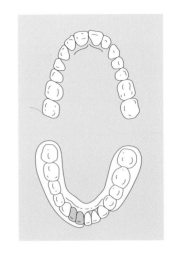

Patient: 70 years old, female

Chief complaint: Fracture of pre-existing denture

Remaining teeth: 13–17, 22–27, 32, 33, 41, 42

Location of magnetic attachments: 41–43

Reasons for use of magnetic attachments: Adequate retention and gaining favorable crown-root ratio

Initial Situation

The patient referred to the clinic with her broken lower denture. The denture was broken around 42 tooth area. The 41, 43 tooth had root copings and 42 tooth was restored by crown. The insufficient thickness of denture base near 42 tooth area was thought to be the reason of the fracture. As the fragments of denture could be fitted precisely and it was made just 2 years ago, the repair of the denture was indicated. The 42 tooth had periapical lesion (*Fig 1*) and showed increased mobility.

Treatment Planning and Procedures

In order to preserve 42 abutment tooth, strengthen the denture base and increase retention, the design of overlaying 41, 42, 43 teeth and application of magnetic attachments were needed to be selected. The crown with post-core was removed from 42 tooth and root copings from 41, 43 teeth. The 41, 42, 43 teeth were prepared and the silicone-rubber impression was taken. Root caps with cast-bonded keepers Hicorex Slim 3013 were fabricated (*Fig 2*) and cemented on 41, 42, 43 abutments. Three magnetic attachments in this case were not necessary, but because of unfavorable prognosis of abutments, keepers were cast-bonded to all root caps in order to make easier repair of the denture if one of the abutments would fail. The denture was relined and repaired and only one magnetic assembly embedded into denture base (*Fig 3*). The occlusion scheme applied in this case was group function occlusion. Patient was instructed on keeping the remaining teeth and denture cleaned.

Outcome of Treatment

Every 3-month patient was recalled for follow-up visit and teeth scaling and minor occlusal

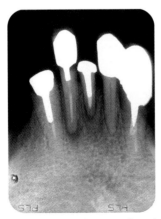

Fig 1 X-ray photo of the lower 41, 42, 43. The periodontal conditions of them were not good especially on the 42 tooth.

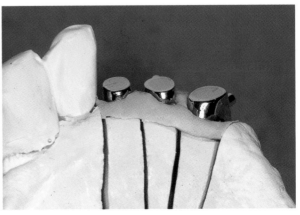

Fig 2 Metal caps with cast-bonded keepers on the working model.

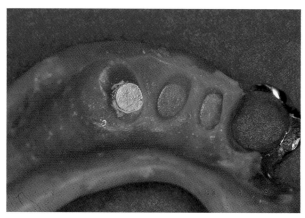

Fig3 The repaired and relined pre-existing denture. Only one magnet was enough to retain the denture.

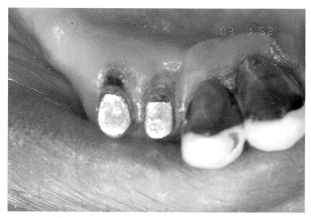

Fig4 Occlusal view of the abutment teeth 3 years after denture relining. The 43 abutment tooth had been extracted because of its fracture.

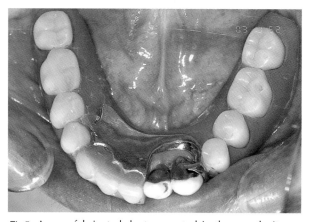

Fig5 A new fabricated denture seated in the mouth. It was reinforced with metal frame.

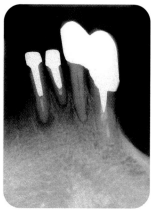

Fig6 X-ray photo of the lower 41, 42 3.5 years after these metal caps were set in the mouth. Stabilized periapical lesions could be observed.

adjustments were performed. Three years after denture relining, patient addressed the clinic complaining about pain of 43 abutment. The clinical and radiological examinations revealed vertical root fracture and thus the 43 tooth was extracted (*Fig4*). Afterwards it was decided to make a new partial overdenture reinforced with metal frame and retained by magnetic attachments on the teeth 41, 42. As the keepers on root caps were already present, the treatment proce-

dure was limited only to fabricating of new metal-framed partial overdenture and embedding magnetic assemblies corresponding with present keepers by auto polymerizing resin (*Fig5*). Three and half years of the first denture setting, the preservation of alveolar bone, proper marginal fit and stabilized periapical lesions could be observed on radiograph of abutments (*Fig6*).

(Hiroshi Mizutani／Vygandas Rutkunas)

Case 9
Improvement of Poor Retention of Lower Denture—2

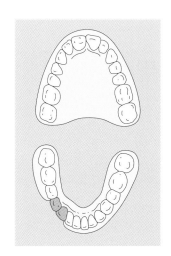

Patient: 70 years old, female

Chief complaints: Poor retention of the upper and lower dentures and difficulty of chewing.

Remaining teeth: 13, 35, 37, 43, 44

Location of magnetic attachments: 43, 44

Reasons for use of magnetic attachments: Improvement of denture retention, and recovery of occlusal relationship

Initial Situation

The patient had full upper and partial lower dentures which were made about five years ago. The dentures were lacking for stability and retention, and the occlusal relationship was greatly disrupted. The patient complained of pain in chewing. Almost all the teeth were involved in caries and moved with periodontal disease.

Treatment Plan and Procedures

First of all, improvement of the dentures was needed so that the patient could chew without pain. The dentures were corrected for the stability under the existing oral conditions though the occlusal relationship was disrupted. After that, tentative dentures were to be made for seeking for suitable occlusal position and preparing oral circumstance for new real dentures. Extraction of disabled teeth and treatment of the residual tissues were performed.

As the result, the upper jaw became edentulous and only the teeth 43, 44 remained in the lower jaw. These were treated for the abutment of removable partial denture (*Fig1*). They were not always in good condition (*Fig2*), but they were expected to be helpful for recovering disturbed occlusal relationship even in a short period.

Magnetic attachments Magfit EX600, 600w

were to be used as the retainer. The keepers were fixed to the abutment teeth 43, 44 (*Fig3*), and the magnets were temporary set in the lower tentative denture.

About one year later, new real dentures were fabricated (*Fig4*). After one month, as the denture was settled down and occlusal relationship was secured (*Fig5*), the magnets in the lower tentative denture were taken off and transferred to the new denture (*Fig6*). No problem was observed with the abutments (*Figs7, 8*). Every six months after setting of the denture, examination and adjustment were performed with the abutments and dentures (*Figs9, 10*).

Outcome of Treatment

After two years, the lower denture was cracked at the lingual part of the abutment and the magnets were shed. The denture was repaired and the magnets were reset. At the present of five years since the new denture was fabricated, there is no problem. The mobility of the teeth 43, 44 was nearly the same as in the beginning. The denture functioned well and the patient was satisfied with it.

The initial oral situation of this patient was miserable with poor fitness of dentures, unstable occlusal relationship, spread of caries and mobility of remaining teeth. Occlusal reconstruction with complete dentures after removing all the teeth might have been proper, but considering the age of the patient, instability of her jaw and distrust against dental treatments, the lines that the teeth

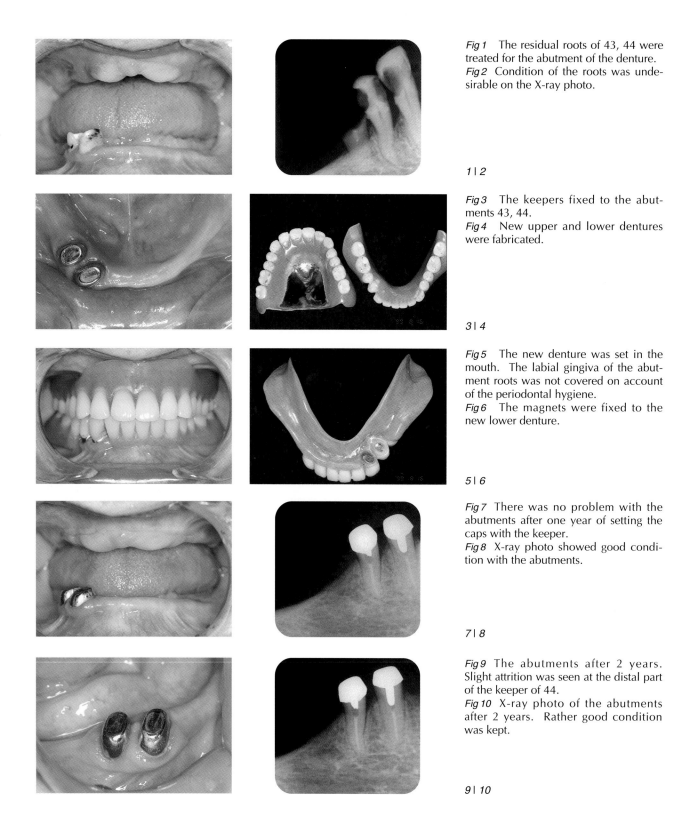

Fig 1 The residual roots of 43, 44 were treated for the abutment of the denture.
Fig 2 Condition of the roots was undesirable on the X-ray photo.

1 | 2

Fig 3 The keepers fixed to the abutments 43, 44.
Fig 4 New upper and lower dentures were fabricated.

3 | 4

Fig 5 The new denture was set in the mouth. The labial gingiva of the abutment roots was not covered on account of the periodontal hygiene.
Fig 6 The magnets were fixed to the new lower denture.

5 | 6

Fig 7 There was no problem with the abutments after one year of setting the caps with the keeper.
Fig 8 X-ray photo showed good condition with the abutments.

7 | 8

Fig 9 The abutments after 2 years. Slight attrition was seen at the distal part of the keeper of 44.
Fig 10 X-ray photo of the abutments after 2 years. Rather good condition was kept.

9 | 10

were preserved as much as possible were chosen.

The teeth 43, 44 which looked doubtful in its preservation at the beginning were keeping good function. This is thought such that excessive load was avoided or adequate functional force acted on the teeth by using magnetic attachments.

In this case the root caps with the keeper were made about 4mm above the margin of the gingiva. This is because of easiness of brushing around the roots. Tall root cap is apt to make the denture unstable because it acts as a fulcrum. But, this can be corrected by regular maintenance.

(Seiichiro Someya)

Case 10
Application after Extrusion of Abutment Root

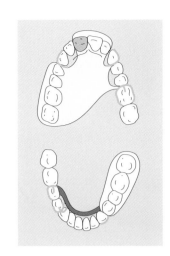

Patient: 65 years old, female

Chief complaints: Loss of a crown of 11 and poor appearance

Remaining teeth: 11–13, 23–27, 31–33, 41–47

Location of magnetic attachments: 11

Reason for use of magnetic attachment: Short root length

Initial Situation

The patient complained of poor appearance due to detachment of an artificial crown.

A crown and metal core of tooth 11 was lost and the root surface of 11 was softened because of dental caries (*Fig 1*). The condition of the bone around 11 was good, but the remaining root was short (*Fig 2*). After removing a carious dentin, upper surface of the root was calculated to be deep under the gingival margin. The maxillary arch was restored with removable partial denture. The patient had a heart disease and her attending physician advised against extraction of the tooth.

Treatment Planning and Procedures

11 was planned to be extruded using a pair of magnets. After infected dentin was removed and sane dentin came over the gingival margin, the root was to serve as an abutment for magnetic overdenture. It was expended to provide periodontal support and minimum but sufficient retention for the denture.

In order to extrude the tooth, a pair of Sm-Co5 magnets (3ø×2mm) was used. They had an attractive force of 30gf when they stayed 1.5mm away from each other. The root canal was prepared for a temporally post. The post was made of autopolymerizing resin and a magnet was mounted in it(*Fig 3*). An artificial tooth of 11 was added to the existing denture, and a hole was made at the bottom of the artificial tooth for a other magnet (*Fig 4*). A piece of paraffin wax with thickness of 1.5mm was placed on the temporally post. Then, another magnet which was to attract to the magnet in the post, was placed on the wax. (*Fig 5*). The hole of the artificial tooth was filled with autopolymerizing resin and placed onto the magnet. After resin cured, the wax was removed the from denture and trimmed it (*Fig 6*). The root was pulled up by attractive force of two magnets. After two weeks, magnets come to attach each other. The root was extruded. Then the temporary post was removed and carious dentin was eliminated. These extruding procedures were repeated until sound dentin came over the gingival margin (*Fig 7*). Finally, the root was retained by using the two magnets until surrounding bone was reconstructed. After 2 month, the root cap with magnetic keeper was cemented to the root (*Fig 8*) and new denture with magnet assembly was inserted (*Fig 9, 10*). The patient had a heart disease and was taking anticoagulant. Her gingiva was inflamed. As 11 was located lingual, gingival margin of the root was completely covered with the denture. This aggravated the inflammation in 11. Brushing of 11 was done well, but the gingiva was still inflamed.

Outcome of Treatment

After 4 years, gingiva was still a little inflamed

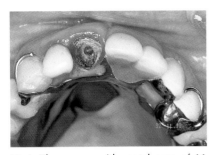

Fig 1 The crown with metal core of 11 was left out. The surface of the root was softened because of dental caries.

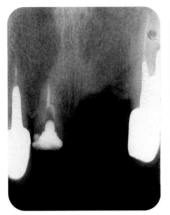
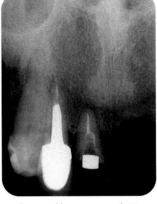

Fig 2 Left: Before extrusion. The condition of bone around 11 was good, but remaining root length was short. Right: After extrusion. 11 was extruded and sound dentin was at suprabony position.

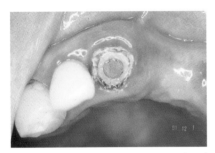

Fig 3 The temporary post was made of autopolymerizing resin and a magnet was mounted in it.

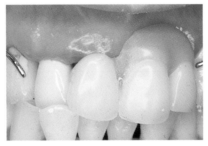

Fig 4 An artificial tooth was added to the existing denture, and holed from the bottom for a magnet.

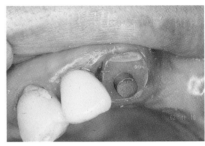

Fig 5 Another magnet, which attracted to the magnet in the post, was placed on the wax.

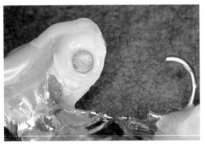

Fig 6 Magnet was mounted in the denture. The root and the denture were attracted each other by the magnets.

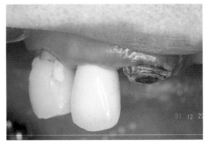

Fig 7 The root was extruded.

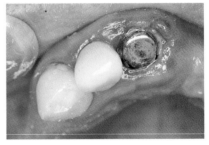

Fig 8 The root cap with magnetic keeper was mounted. Gingiva around the root was still inflamed.

9 | 10

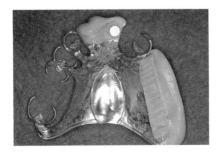
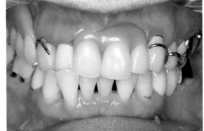

Fig 9 The denture completely covered the root cap. Metal framework was opened around the magnetic assembly.
Fig 10 Frontal view. Labial denture border of 11 was kept minimum coverage.

(Fig 11), but the mobility of 11 was not increased and surrounding bone was not receding. The surface of the magnetic assembly was not worn (Fig 12).

After 6 years, 34 and 36 were extracted at the attending hospital because of the fracture of the bridge and its abutment roots. 26 and 27 were damaged too. At this time, 24–27 were restored

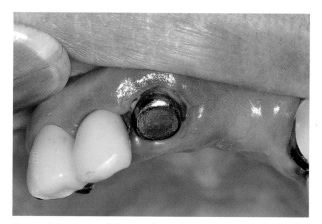

Fig 11 11 remained in good condition. Gingiva was still a little inflamed.

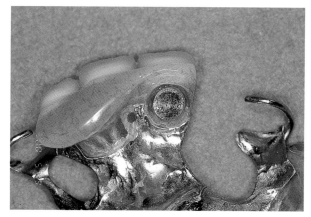

Fig 12 Magnetic assembly and surrounding resin were in good condition. Attractive force of the magnet kept its default value.

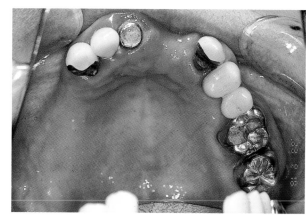

Fig 13-15 New partial denture.

	13
14	15

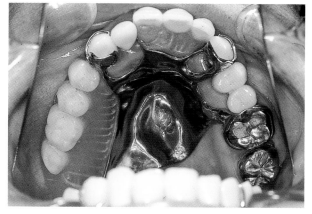

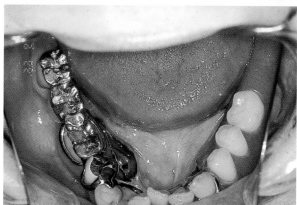

with the bridge and other missing teeth were restored with partial dentures. 11 was used as a magnetic retainer again (*Fig 13–15*).

Now, 9 years has past, 11 is kept in good condition and the magnetic assembly has kept it shine.

Only the magnetic attachment can keep such poor tooth in useful and healthy condition.

(Kazuo Nakamura)

Case 11
Application for Short Length Root—1

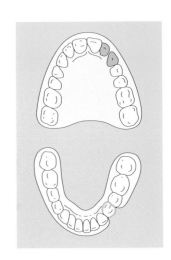

Patient: 70 years old, female

Chief complaint: Instability of the upper denture due to loss of the crown of 13

Remaining teeth: 11, 21–23, 31, 34, 35, 41

Location of magnetic attachments: 23

Reason for use of magnetic attachment: short root length

Initial Situation

The patient complained of instability, poor retention of the upper denture after loss of abutment canine. The remaining teeth were in good periodontal condition, but because of bone resorption their crown-root ratios were large (*Fig 1*). There were deep wedge-shaped defects and proximal caries on 22 and 23. The crown of 22 was cracked at the wedge-shaped defect. After endodontic treatments, 22 was filled with composite resin and 23 was cut at the height of gingiva. The patient wore one-piece cast partial denture with cast rests and wire clasps on 11 and 23.

Treatment Planning and Procedures

In order to reduce the crown-root ratio, 22 and 23 were to be used as the root capped abutment. After endodontic treatment, 22 was filled with resin and the root cap with magnetic keeper was applied to only 23. It was expected that these roots provided enough periodontal support for the denture and the magnetic attachment application on 23 enables the denture to obtain good retention. Cast rest and wire clasp was applied to 11.

The diameter of the root surface of 22 was shorter than that of existing magnetic keeper. 22 was not in good condition with mobility, so its root surface was to be tentatively filled with composite resin. Artificial teeth of 22 and 23 were added to the existing denture. The keeper of the magnetic attachment Hicolex MD was applied for 23 (*Fig 2*).

The root surface of 23 was prepared parallel to the occlusal plane. The root notably exposed its buccal surface due to gingival recession. After cementing the root cap, magnetic assembly coated with metal adhesive resin Super-Bond was embedded in the denture with autopolymerizing resin (*Fig 3*). The denture border was adjust a little beneath the gingival margins at 22, but above the gingival margin at 23 because of the undercut area (*Fig 4*).

Outcome of Treatment

After 4 years, 41, 31 and 34 were extracted because of periodontitis. Then, upper and lower dentures were renewed. After recovery from the wound, impression for the denture was made. Stone replicas of the magnetic assemblies were mounted on the root caps of the master cast. The portions of the retentive framework over the root caps were opened to leave room for the magnetic assemblies, but the framework was reinforced around the root cap (*Fig 5–7*).

After a year, 21 came off, but 22 kept good condition. At this time a smaller keeper appeared in the market. So the application of magnetic retainer was planned to the tooth 22. 22 was prepared for the root cap with magnetic keeper and artificial tooth of 21 was added to the denture (*Fig 8*).

After a year, 11 finally came off and the denture had to be changed to the complete magnetic overdenture. With the passing of 4 years, this

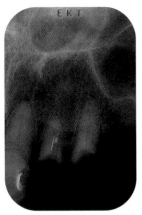

Fig 1 Because of bone resorption crown-root ratios were large.

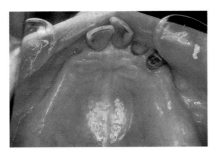

Fig 2 Occlusal view of maxilla. 22 was filled with resin. Magnetic keeper was mounted on 23.

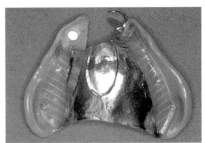

Fig 3 Artificial teeth were added to the denture and magnetic assembly was embedded in it.

Fig 4 Frontal view. Buccal surfaces of the anterior teeth were widely exposed. Denture border was beneath the gingival margin of the root cap.

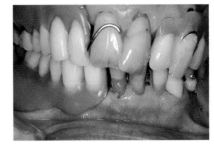

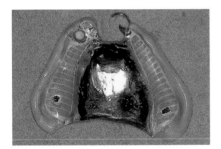

Fig 5 New denture. The metal framework around the magnet assembly was reinforced. The denture gave space to the magnetic assembly.

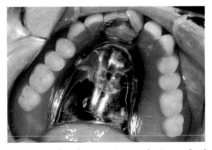

Fig 6 Occlusal view. Lingual gingival of 11 and 21 was opened.

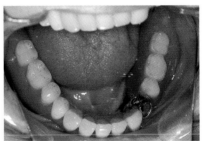

Fig 7 Mandibular new denture. 41, 31, 34 were lost and 35 was restored with metal crown.

8 | 9

Fig 8 After 21 came off, 22 was restored with root cap with magnetic keeper. Magnetic assembly coated with metal adhesive resin attached on the magnetic keeper of 22.

Fig 9 Finally, 11 was lost and only the root caps remained.

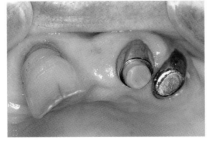

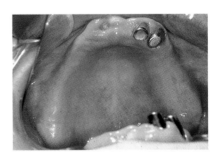

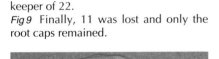

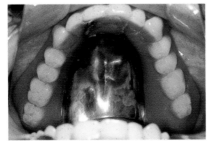

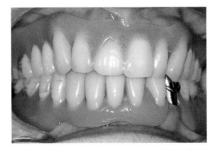

Fig 10–12 Complete magnetic overdenture shows good result.

10 | 11 | 12

denture works well now (Fig 9–12).

Magnetic attachment system improves crown-root ratio and avoids damaging lateral and rotating forces from the denture. Magnetic attachment system may be the best retainer for the teeth under unfavorable conditions.

(Kazuo Nakamura)

Case 12
Application for Short Length Root—2

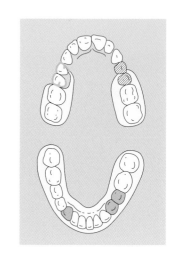

Patient: 66 years old, female

Chief complaint: Difficulty of chewing function because of the damaged bridge

Remaining teeth: 11−17, 21−26, 33−35, 42, 43

Location of magnetic attachments: 34, 35, 43

Reason for use of magnetic attachments: short root length

Initial Sistuation

The patient complained of difficulty of chewing due to damage of the lower anterior bridge. Treatment teeth 42, 43 and 33 were decayed at the margin of crowns (*Fig1,2*). The remaining teeth had severe worn occlusal surfaces and their neighboring gingiva was swollen and bleeding. Especially 42 and 33 were heavily decayed and had swollen gingiva. Other lower teeth were loose with short roots. These findings suggested that the restoration using fixed bridge was not indicated. All the upper teeth were restored and fastened with fixed bridge and their occlusal surfaces were heavily worn (*Fig3*).

Treatment Planning and Procedures

Broken bridge was removed. As 42 and 33 were too poor to be kept, they were extracted. Remaining teeth 43, 34, and 35 were applied to abutments. In order to reduce the crown-root ratio, they were used as the root capped teeth with magnetic keepers (*Fig4,5*). It was expected that these roots provided periodontal support for the denture, while the retention was provided by the magnetic attachment system on remaining roots.

Before removing the lower bridge, impression for the immediate complete denture was made. 42 and 33 were extracted following the removal of the fixed partial denture. 43, 34 and 35 were decoronated and prepared for the root caps (*Fig6*). Gum contour of the teeth was duplicated with silicone impression material (*Fig7*). In making wax patterns of the root caps, wax around the keeper was contoured wider than the desired form to prevent the error of casting, and they were trimmed after cast. Upper surfaces of these root caps were prepared parallel to the occlusal plane and the attractive surfaces of the keepers cast on them were aligned (*Fig8*). The lower immediate denture was inserted onto the root caps. Then it was trimmed and holed to leave room for the magnetic assemblies. Magnetic assemblies coated with metal adhesive resin Super-Bond were mounted in the denture with autopolymerizing resin (*Fig9,10*). As the root caps were completely covered with the denture, patient was instructed to brush remaining roots and to have a periodic check-up. The denture never lifted even while swimming and the patient was satisfied with it.

Outcome of Treatment

Next year, the upper teeth 26 was lost. At this moment, 11, 12, 21–23 were restored with splinted crowns and 26, 27 were restored with cone telescope crowns (*Fig11*). The patient brushed roots well, but plaque was accumalated at the marginal undercut area of the root caps (*Fig12*). The surrounding bone of 43, 34 and 35 got well(*Fig13,14*).

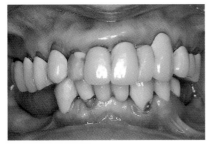

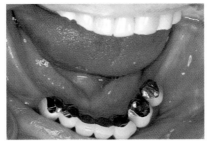

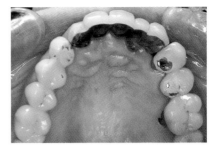

Fig 1,2 The fixed partial denture in mandibule was broken. 42, 43 and 33 were decayed at the margin of crowns.

Fig 3 All the teeth in maxilla were restored and fastened with the fixed partial denture and their occlusal surfaces were heavily worn.

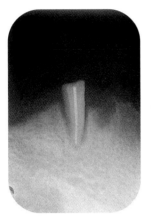

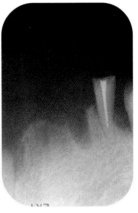

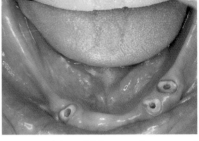

Fig 4,5 Remaining teeth were applied to abutments. They were loose with short roots, too.

Fig 6 43, 34 and 35 were decoronated and prepared for the root caps.

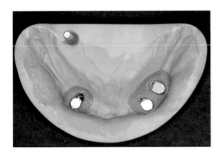

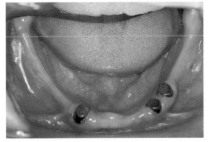

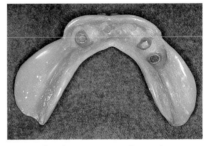

Fig 7 Gum contour was duplicated with silicone impression material.

Fig 8 Occlusal view. the attractive surfaces of the keepers prepared parallel to the occlusal plane.

Fig 9 The lower complete denture. Magnetic assemblies were mounted in the denture with autopolymerizing resin.

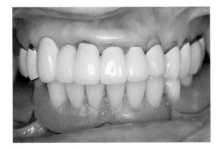

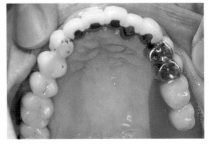

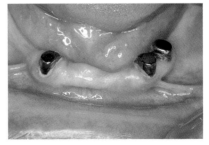

Fig 10 Frontal view.

Fig 11 12–23 were restored with splinted crowns and 26,27 were restored with cone telescope crowns.

Fig 12 Even she brushed roots well, there were plaque at the marginal undercut area of the root caps.

After another year, 17 was lost. 13–15 were restored with crowns and 16, 17 were restored with a removable partial denture (Fig 15).

The magnetic assembly used here was a bit higher and wider, and the lingual of the denture was a little bulged surface at the magnetic assemblies. This was the only one problem for the patient. At this time, smaller magnetic assemblies Hicolex Super-J3515 could be obtained. Then, a new overdenture was to be made using this.

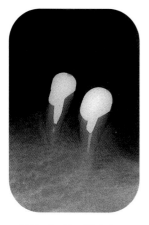
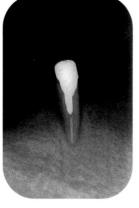
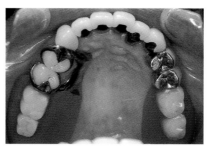

Fig 13,14 The surrounding bone got well.
Fig 15 13–15 were restored with crowns and 16,17 were restored with a removable partial denture.

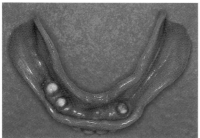

Fig 16 New denture. Stone replicas could leave minimum room for the magnetic assembly in the denture.

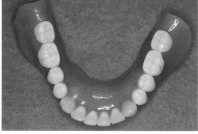

Fig 17 New denture had a correct lingual coutour.

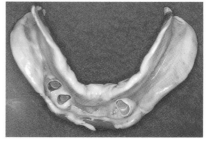

Fig 18 Magnetic assemblies and the denture were well-adapt to the root caps and the ridge.

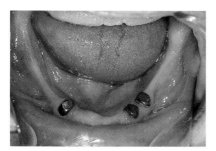

Fig 19 Roots were a little exposed but their surfaces were kept clean.

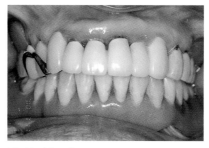

Fig 20 After 6 years, crowns, root caps and dentures had a good prognosis.

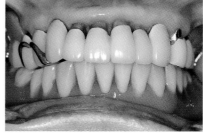

Fig 21 After 10 years, remaining bone was resorbed and roots were exposed because of her systemic disease.

22 | 23

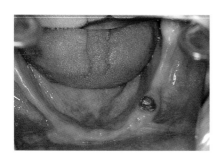
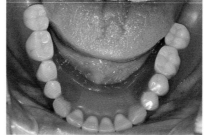

Fig 22,23 43 and 34 were lost. But the denture still works well enough.

Before arrangement of artificial teeth and wax-up, stone replicas of the magnetic assemblies were mounted on the root caps of the master cast.

This could leave minimum room for the magnetic assembly (*Fig 16*). The denture could be made with correct lingual coutour (*Fig 17*).

After 6 years, root caps and the denture showed a good outcome. The roots were a little exposed but their surfaces were kept clean (*Fig 18–20*).

After 10 years, the remaining bone was considerably resorbed and roots were exposed because of her systemic disease. 43 and 34 were lost. But the denture still works well enough (*Fig 21–23*).

(Kazuo Nakamura)

Case 13
Application for Abutment with Reduced Periodontal Support

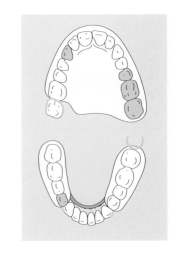

Patient: 58 years old, female

Chief complaints: Fracture of upper and lower abutment teeth, loss of denture retention and stability

Remaining teeth: 13, 17, 25–27, 31–33, 38, 41–43

Location of magnetic attachments: 13, 25, 27, 44

Reason for use of magnetic attachments: Preservotion of reduced periodontal support of abutments

Initial Situation

The patient complained of broken upper and lower abutment teeth and of resulted lost retention of her dentures. 13 and 44 abutment teeth were broken and needed to be restored as well as to make a new dentures in order to restore and maintain vertical dimension (*Fig1a–c*). The periodontal condition of 13, 25–27 and 44 roots were evaluated by radiographs (*Fig2a–c*). The root canal of 44 tooth was not filled fully; the root was retreated (*Fig3*). The lower anterior teeth were splinted by composite resin (*Fig1a*).

Treatment Planning and Procedure

The root caps with cast-bonded keepers were fabricated and cemented on 13, 25, 27 and 44. Hyperslim 3513 for 13, Hyperslim 3013 for 27 and Magfit 400 for 25 and 44 were selected.

New dentures were made and magnetic assemblies were embedded in denture base with auto polymerizing acrylic resin. Because of compromised periodontal status of upper teeth and decreased ability to provide support, the complete palatal coverage in design of upper denture was chosen. 38 tooth was in infraocclusal position and the cap clasp crown as a retention device was used. Support in anterior region of lower was gained from occlusal rests on 33, 43 and retention was balanced with I bar on the left side. Cleaning of denture and remaining teeth with restorations was emphasized and schedule for follow-up appointments was set.

Outcome of Treatment

Two years after treatment, the root caps remained without complications (*Fig4a,b*). Patient didn't have any complains about loss of retention and/or stability in the stage of two and a half years. (*Fig5a–c*). Decrease in magnetic

Fig 1a–c Dental condition upon presentation.

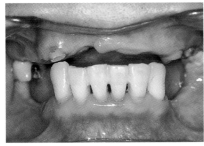

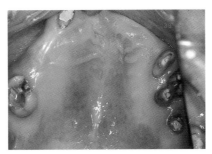

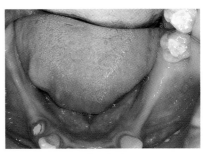

Fig 1a Frontal view. No occlusal contacts between upper and lower natural teeth.

Fig 1b Upper occlusal view. 26, 27 were hemi sectioned.

Fig 1c Lower occlusal view

Fig 2a–c X-ray photos upon presentation.

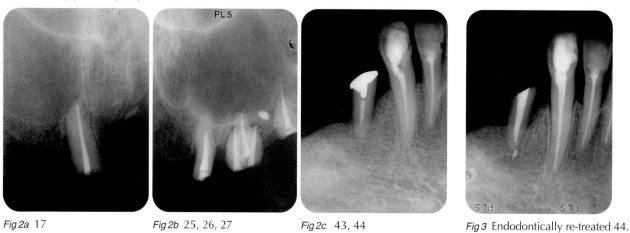

Fig 2a 17

Fig 2b 25, 26, 27

Fig 2c 43, 44

Fig 3 Endodontically re-treated 44.

Fig 4a, b Oral cavities one and a half years after the new dentures were set in the mouth.

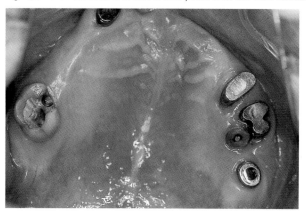

Fig 4a Upper occlusal view.

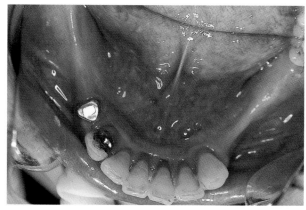

Fig 4b Lower occlusal view.

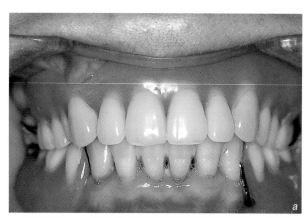

Fig 5a–c The condition of the mouth after 2 years after the denture setting.

Fig 5a Frontal view. I-bar clasp was applied on the 33 abutment tooth.
Fig 5b Upper occlusal view.
Fig 5c Lower occlusal view.

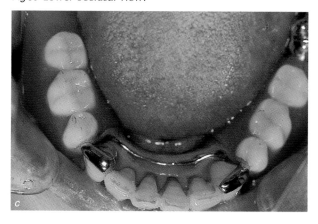

Fig 6a, b X-ray photos five years after the the denture setting.

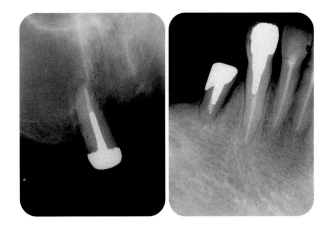

a | b

Fig 6a 13 abutment tooth. Alveolar bone around the abutment has shown slight resorption compared to "before treatment stage".
Fig 6b 44 abutment tooth. Alveolar bone in the medial side has shown remarkable bone resorption but almost the same compared to the "before treatment stage".

attractive forces or other signs of corrosion (discoloration, deformation of magnetic assembly etc.) or scratching of keeper surface after 4 years were insignificant. However in x-ray photos of 33 and 44 abutments after 5 years the slight resorption of periapical bone was seen (*Fig 6a, b*).

(Hiroshi Mizutani／Vygandas Rutkunas)

Case 14
Application for a Fractured Tooth

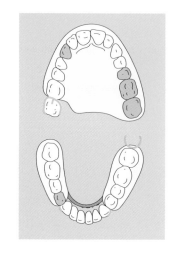

Patient: 62 years old, female

Chief complaints: Fracture of abutment tooth and loss of denture retention

Remaining teeth: 13, 23–25, 31–34, 41–44

Location of magnetic attachments: 44

Reason for use of magnetic attachments: Ease of application, preservation of periodontium, adequate retention and stability

Initial Situation

The patient referred to clinic complaining of fractured tooth and lost retention of lower denture. The first right lower premolar was broken and the retention of stability of lower RPD was eventually lost. The quality of upper and lower RPDs were adequate, thus remaking of dentures was rejected. The 44 root was suitable as an abutment (*Fig2*). Owing to ease of application and relevant retentive properties, the application of magnetic attachment was selected. Thus complicated procedure of making a new crown fitting to the pre-existing clasp was avoided.

Treatment Planning and Procedure

The shape of root cross-section dictated selection of oval form Magfit with retentive force of 600 gf. During wax-up of root cap the keeper was attached and cast-bonded during casting. For casting root cap the gold-palladium alloy was used. After polishing the root cap with keeper attached was cemented (*Fig3a*). The artificial tooth was set in the place of missing 44 and magnetic assembly was embedded into denture base by means of auto polymerizing resin (*Fig3b*). The proper retention and stability of dentures were regained and the patient reported comfortable wearing and chewing and improved esthetics as well. She was instructed about the maintenance and follow-up visits.

Outcome of Treatment

After 4 and a half years, root cap on 44 remained in good condition: no caries or signs of crevice corrosion were noticeable (*Fig4*). After 10 years of observation, retention of dentures was unchanged and there were no signs of corrosion. Due to adequate hygiene periodontal tissues around keeper remained healthy (*Fig5a*) and post-treatment care was limited to relining and

1|2

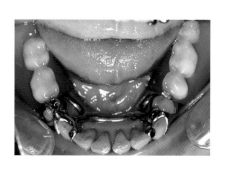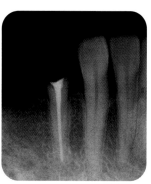

Fig 1 Occlusal view of lower 1 year before 44 was fractured.
Fig 2 An x-ray photo immediately after the fracture of 44.

Fig 3a, b A metal cap with keeper was set and an artificial tooth with the magnet was added in the former denture.

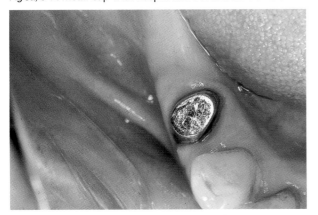

Fig 3a Metal cap with keeper immediately after cementation.

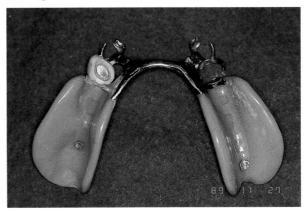

Fig 3b The former denture with magnet.

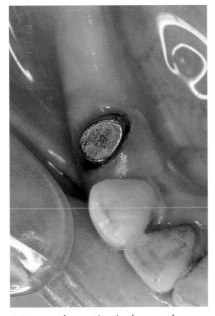

Fig 4 The metal cap 4.5 years after setting in the mouth.

Fig 5a, b Ten years after the denture setting.

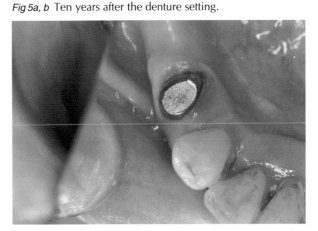

Fig 5a The gingiva around the metal cap kept being healthy. No signs of corrosion and inflammation was observed.

occlusal adjustments (*Fig 3b*). Twelve years after the end of treatment, since the upper RPD and lower partial overdenture underwent excessive wear of artificial teeth, particularly 44 and unstability of the denture bases, new metal framed dentures were fabricated (*Fig 6a–c*). During this period keeper underwent minor changes as slight scratching without any clinically detectable influence on retention and stability. Any signs of corrosion of casting-keeper interface were not detected, thus the new lower overdenture was constructed with old keeper remaining (*Fig 6d*). Both professional and personal hygiene procedures seemed to be adequate. Denture status and

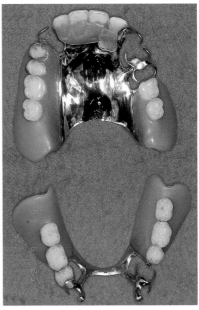

Fig 5b Upper and lower dentures. Wears of artificial teeth were observed.

Fig 6a–d Twelve years after initial treatment. New metal framed dentures were fabricated.

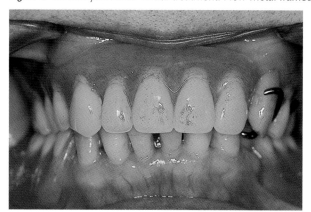

Fig 6a The dentures were set in the mouth.

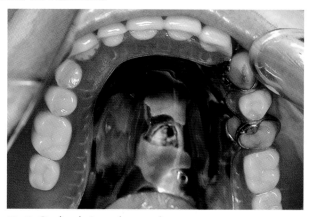

Fig 6b Occlusal view of upper denture.

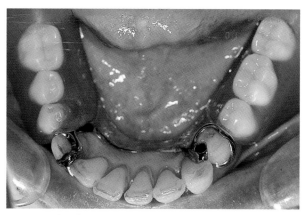

Fig 6c Occlusal view of lower denture.

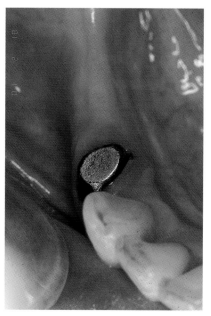

Fig 6d Metal cap with keeper in the mouth. No inflammation was observed and healthy.

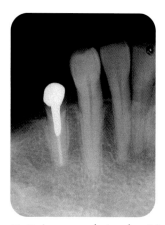

Fig 7 An x-ray photo after 14 years after initial treatment. The volume of alveolar bone around the abutment was still eoungh.

oral health 14 years after treatment were well preserved, besides patient satisfaction was high and magnetic attachment kept retentive properties unchanged. Slight bone resorption around 44 could be seen in the radiograph after 14 years of service, thus suggesting that magnetic attachments have high capability to preserve abutment health (*Fig 7*).

(Hiroshi Mizutani／Vygandas Rutkunas)

Case 15
Application Together with Root Surface Attachment

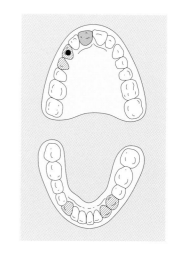

Patient: 57 years old, male

Chief complaints: Dysfunction of mastication and instability of prosthetic appliances.

Remaining teeth: 11–15, 17, 21–24, 33, 34, 43

Location of magnetic attachments: 11

Reason for use of magnetic attachments: Path direction difference between denture insertion and middle incisor roots and improvement of esthetical unappealing.

Initial Situation

The patient addressed the clinic with complaint of masticatory dysfunction and instability of dentures. The dentition and prosthetic appliances were highly damaged (*Fig 1a, b*). Upper teeth were restored by fixed dentures whose fit was bad and they were worn out. Hygiene was insufficient and therefore accumulation of plaque resulted in periodontitis and consequent increased mobility. Radiographs of upper teeth (*Fig 2a, b*) confirmed advanced periodontitis and considerable bone loss.

Treatment Planning and Procedure

Thus, according to above-mentioned clinical and radiological findings, the upper 12, 15, 17, 21–24 teeth were subjected to extractions. The 11, 13 teeth were prepared for root cap and,

since the coronal part of 14 tooth was not damaged by caries significantly, it was prepared for cast coping (*Fig 3*). As the direction of 11 did not conform to the insertion path, it was decided to apply magnetic attachment on the tooth. The Hicorex 4013 was applied on 11 teeth. The directions of 13, 14 teeth were judged to coincide with path of insertion. It enabled to apply cylindrical Dalla Bona to 13, Type IV gold alloy cast coping to 14 and Pd-Ag-Au alloy root cap with cast bonded keeper to 11 teeth. The new upper and lower overdentures were fabricated and inserted (*Fig 4*). The lower overdenture was retained by conic crowns on 33, 34, 43 teeth. Patient was educated to clean the teeth and dentures. Personal and professional hygiene were emphasized.

Outcome of Treatment

Two years after the denture setting, magnetic assembly remained firmly embedded into denture acrylic base and the surface of neither it or keeper were scratched (*Fig 5*). The mechanical

Fig 1a, b Dental condition upon presentation. Advanced caries and periodontitis were observed.

a | b

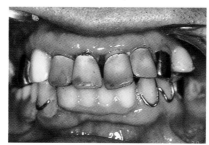 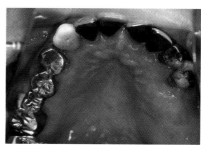

Fig 1a Frontal view of the mouth.
Fig 1b Upper occlusal view.

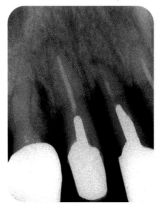

Fig 2a 13, 14

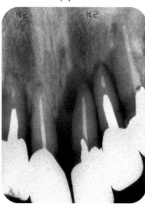

Fig 2b 11, 12, 21, 22

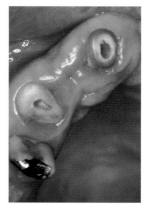

Fig 3 Prepared 11, 13, 14 teeth. 14 tooth was prepared for conic crown because not damaged so much.

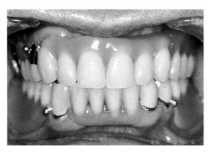

Fig 4 Frontal view of the mouth immediately after new denture insertion.

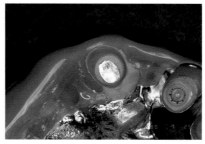

Fig 5 The keeper embedded in the denture 2 years after the denture setting.

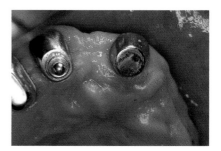

Fig 6 The keeper and the Dalla Bona male attachment 4 years after the denture setting. Mucosa around the abutments looked healthy.

Fig 8 The keeper and the Dalla Bona male attachment 13 years after the denture setting. No signs of corrosion of magnetic assembly were observed.

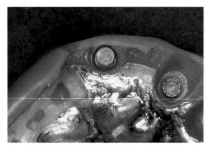

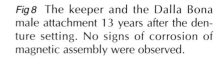

7 | 8

Fig 7 The magnetic assembly and the Dalla Bona female attachment 9 years after the denture setting. The magnet was the same one as the pre-used, while the Dalla Bona female and outer cap of 14 conic crown were changed because of fracture.

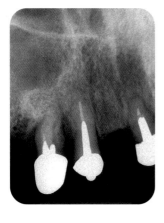

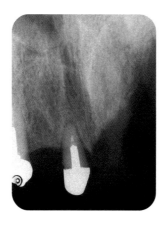

Fig 9a, b X-ray photos of upper 13, 14, 21 teeth 14.5 years after the denture setting. Vertical bone resorption was recognized on every abutment, but slightly compared to the 'upon presentation stage' (Fig2B, Fig2C).

a | b

Fig 9a 13, 14 teeth.
Fig 9b 11 tooth.

Fig 10a–c Dental conditions 15 years after the denture setting. The periodontal conditions were not so bad though there had not been natural teeth contacts between upper and lower jaw. The root caps of the 11, 13 and the inner caps of the 14 and the 33, 34 have never been detached from the abutments during this 15 years period.

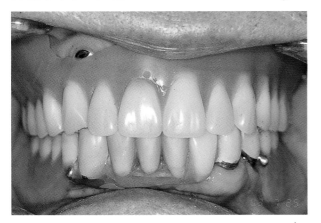

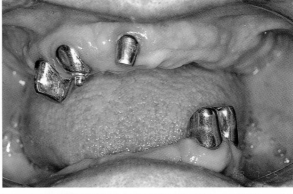

a	b
	c

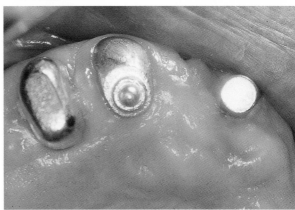

Fig 10a Frontal view of the mouth with the dentures.
Fig 10b Frontal view of the mouth without the dentures.
Fig 10c Occlusal view of the upper abutments.

Dalla Bona and cast coping remained in proper condition. Four years (*Fig 6*), 9 years (*Fig 7*) and 13 years (*Fig 8*) after the denture insertion, even though magnetic attachment underwent minor changes, it provided required retention and stability. However Dalla Bona female had to be replaced after 9 years of use. The upper and lower dentures were relined twice and patient ensured adequate hygiene of the dentures and abutments throughout this period. The radiographs fourteen and half years after the denture setting showed no signs of secondary caries and vertical alveolar bone resorption was insignificant

(*Fig 9a, b*). Fifteen years after the denture setting, all upper abutments remained in proper condition (*Fig 10a*) with good marginal fit, healthy periodontal tissues and adequate retention and stability. The 43 abutment was lost (*Fig 10b, c*) due to progressed bone resorption and lower overdenture was relined in this place by auto-polymerizing resin. As occlusion of overdentures was corrected just slightly and fitting of bases ensured by relining, the patient continued to use overdentures and was satisfied with them.

(Hiroshi Mizutani／Vygandas Rutkunas)

Case 16
Application together with Telescope Crowns

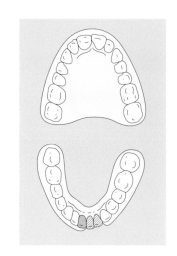

Patient: 32 years old, female

Chief complaint: Masticatory disorder

Remaining teeth: 31–33, 41, 42

Location of magnetic attachments: 41

Reasons for use of magnetic attachments: Reinforcement of denture retention

Initial Situation

This lady came with complaint of masticatory disorder with poor stability and retention of upper complete denture without lower dental restoration. She lost almost of all her teeth due to generalized periodontal disease for years. She consulted to her house dentist, if she could restore her masticatory performance and esthetics at the same time. The house dentist introduced her to our university clinic.

Upper complete denture had nearly lost all stability and retention with discolourated denture resin after recurrent repairs and relininings.

X-ray inspection revealed the poor periodontal support around the remaining lower anterior teeth. Extractions of all remaining teeth were strictly suggested after periodontal examination. (Fig 1, 2)

Treatment Plan and Procedures

Since, she had no experience to wear lower denture for years, tentative treatment denture was first designed to accustom her to wearing dentures and to preserve the lower teeth as abutments if possible. Extensive oral hygiene care was programmed with tooth brushing and mouth rinse by dental hygienist. Temporary lower tissue supported denture was made with continuous labial clasp on the remaining teeth. Upper denture was also relined for the tissue treatment of the underlining mucosa. Extensive periodontal treatment was done in accordance with her adjustment to the dentures (Fig 3, 4).

Improvement of the crown-root ratio of the remaining teeth and associated endodontic treatment were highly suggested, in the course of periodontal treatment. Lower denture was reformed to the complete overdenture, after cutting the clinical crowns of the anterior teeth after healing of the bleeding from the periodontal pockets by probing. This was done after three moths from the initial fabrication of the temporary denture.

In the meantime, lower remaining roots exhibited partly solid periodontal tissue without marked pockets in other teeth (Fig 5).

Reassessment was done if the remaining teeth might serve as abutment for the final over denture after six months from the initial treatment.

Teeth 31, 32 were judged to preserve as telescopic retainers with slight tooth mobility and normal periodontal pocket respectively. Tooth 41 was judged to serve as a root cap retainer with magnetic attachment with slight tooth mobility but remained periodontal fear. Tooth 33 was judged to preserve only as a root cap for supporting element with little periodontal recovery. Retainers and root caps were fabricated with dowel cores in 31, 32 for build ups. The magnetic attachments of oval type Magfit EX 600 was selected with the keeper cast in the root cap of the abutment 41. Mandibular overdenture was

Fig 1 The remaining anteriors exhibited marked tooth mobility to be extracted respectively.

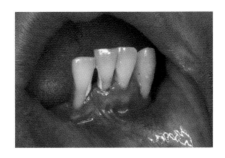

Fig 2 X-ray photo revealed extreme loss of periodontal support of each tooth.

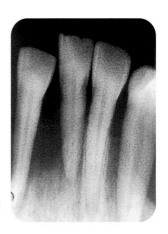

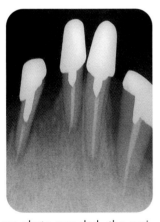

Fig 3 Interim tissue supported RPD with continuous labial clasp was first fabricated for her masticatory recovery.

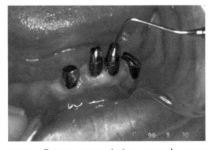

Fig 4 She wore this denture for three months with incorporation to wearing.

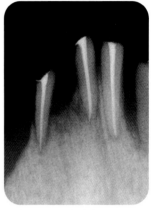

Fig 5 X-ray photo revealed the recovery of the periodontal environment partly around the teeth with devitalization and root canal therapy associated to the improvement of the C R ratio of the remaining teeth.

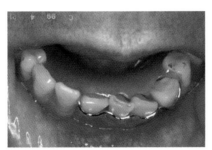

Fig 6 X-ray photo revealed the periodontal status after intensive periodontal treatment and the improvement of the CR ratio of the four anteriors.

Fig 7 Every remaining tooth was judged to select suitable retainer after periodontal reassessment; that means from the telescope retainers on 31, 32, magnetic attachment on 41 and only with metal cap on 33 respectively.

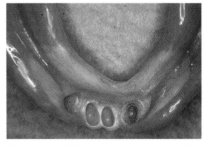

Fig 8 Metal free design reinforced by Targis-Vectoris composite frame resin base denture was first fabricated without the magnetic attachment untill the incorporation of the denture.

made after the conventional clinical procedures. Abutments 31, 32 were telescoped with thin inner conical crowns with the taper of 6 degree respectively. The overdenture was first fabricated without the magnetic attachments. The removable parts of the telescope retainers were made of reinforced plastics Targis-Vectoris without any metal matrix.

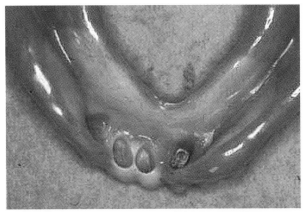

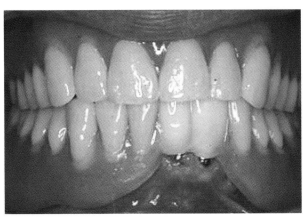

9|10
11|

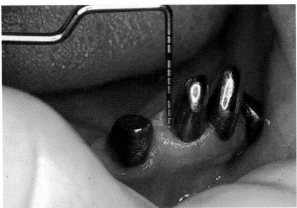

Fig 9 The magnetic attachment Magfit EX 600 was then attached to the overdenture by the self-curing resin.
Fig 10 Favorable esthetic result with patent satisfaction.
Fig 11 Healthy periodontal condition of the abutments has maintained.

The magnetic attachment was then fixed in the lower overdenture after incorporation of the denture. (Fig 6–10)

Outcome of Treatment

Follow-up inspection was executed every six months to support the prosthetic performance and maintain oral health with dentures. She neglected the first appointment after six months and came to our department when the artificial tooth of her upper denture was fallen out 9 moths after the first fabrication.

The prognosis is fairly well. Periodontal condition and mobility of four abutments exhibited not any change in comparison when she first wore this prosthesis.

The magnetic attachment at 41 worked in good function. There was no wear and corrosion observed on the attractive surface of both on the magnetic attachments and keeper (Fig 11).

(Yoshimasa Igarashi)

Case 17
Improvement of Crown-Root Ratio of Abutments—1

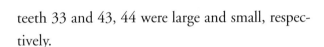

Patient: 85 years old, female

Chief complaint: Dysfunction of mastication due to occlusal imbalance between upper complete overdenture and lower partial denture

Remaining teeth: 33, 42, 43

Location of magnetic attachments: 33, 43, 44

Reason for use of magnetic attachments: Improvement of CR ratio for good retention and stability of lower overdenture.

At the time of the patient's visit, the crown of the abutment teeth 44 had fractured, causing dysfunction of mastication without balance in the lower clasp partial denture supported on the abutment teeth 33, 43, 44. She also complained that the upper complete overdenture was unstable due to long-term use.

Initial Situation

The crowns of the lower remaining tooth 44 had fractured, but the root still existed.

Due to the extrusion of teeth 33, 43 the clinical crown length got longer (*Fig 1*). As shown in panoramic radiography *Fig 2*, alveolar bone resorption in tooth 33 was observed. On the other hand, a slight alveolar bone resorption was shown in teeth 43, 44. Therefore the mobility for

teeth 33 and 43, 44 were large and small, respectively.

Treatment Plan and Procedures

A magnetic attachment-retained overdenture was applied to teeth 33, 43, 44. The reasons for using magnetic attachments in this clinical case were as follows:

The crowns of teeth 33, 43 were long, and from a clinical viewpoint (stress control) it was not suitable to retain the remobable partial denture to the abutment teeth 33, 43 with clasp-retainer.

When dealing with the large mobility of tooth 33, it was necessary to protect the abutment tooth 33 from the lateral stress of the retainer.

In order to avoid Kelly's combination syndrome, (anterior hyperfunction syndrome) which arises from the combination of the upper complete denture and the free-end-partial denture supported on the lower anterior remaining teeth.

In order to modify the existing clasp

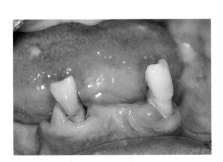

Fig 1 Intra-oral photograph on the patient's first visit.

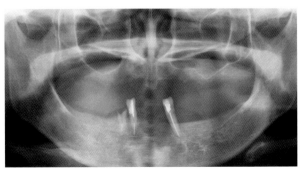

Fig 2 Panoramic radiography.

149

Fig 3 Temporary post crown with the same form as the natural teeth.
Fig 4 Keeper embedded in wax pattern.

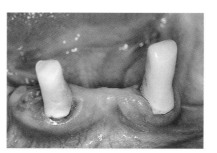

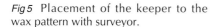
3 | 4

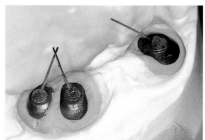

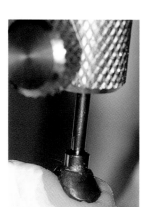

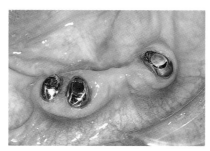

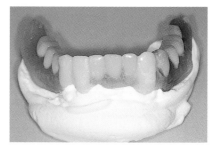

Fig 5 Placement of the keeper to the wax pattern with surveyor.

Fig 6 Cemented root cap incorporated keeper.

Fig 7 Temporary overdenture.

denture as a temporary denture, first, an alginate impression was taken of the region of the lower remaining teeth and the residual ridge. This was because the crowns of teeth 33, 43 would be restored as an existing denture with temporary crown after cutting off the crown parts of the teeth 33, 43. Preparation of the root surface of the teeth 33, 43, 44 was carried out and the pocket was removed by electric surgery. After that, the ready-made metal post was placed into the root canal, the self-curing resin was inserted into the crowns 33, 43 of the alginate impression, and then the impression was placed back in the lower part of the patient's mouth.

After curing the resin, a temporary resin post crown was made. The temporary resin crown was adhered, and then lower existing dentures were used as temporary dentures (Fig 3).

For making a root cap incorporated with keeper and modifying the existing denture, a plaster model was made by taking an impression of the root surface and the root canal. Fig 4 shows that the keepers on the wax pattern are set to be parallel to the occlusal plane.

When placing the keepers on the abutment

teeth, a surveyor tool provides useful assistance (Fig 5). After casting and polishing, the root cap incorporated with the keeper was cemented to the abutment teeth (Fig 6).

The clasps were removed from the existing lower denture and this denture was placed in the patient's mouth. A pickup impression was then taken by using alginate impression materials. On the plaster model, temporary resin crowns were made for the teeth 33, 43 and then adhered to the denture with self-curing resin (Fig 7). This temporary overdenture was used until the final overdentures were completed.

For making the final overdentures, a final impression was taken on the individual tray by using silicone impression materials. The maxillo-mandiblular registration was performed by using bite rim, and the upper and lower plaster models were set on the articulator. The arrangement of the upper and lower artificial teeth was performed with the gypsum dummy of the magnetic assembly adhered to the keeper in the plaster model. (Fig 8, 9)

Polymerization of the upper and lower wax denture was carried out, and after polishing the

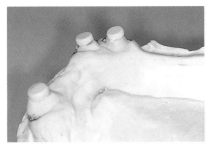

Fig 8 Adhered gypsum dummy on the keeper.

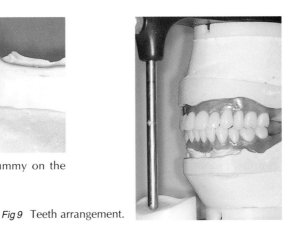

Fig 9 Teeth arrangement.

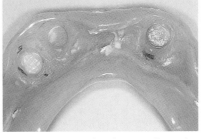

Fig 10 Space in the denture base for magnetic assembly.

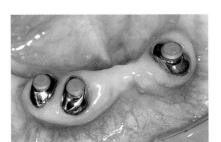

Fig 11 Placement of the magnetic assembly squarely on the keeper.

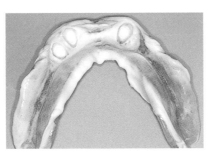

Fig 12 Denture base with fit test material to check the space for magnetic assembly.

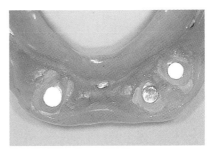

Fig 13 Denture with firmly fixed magnetic assembly.

denture was completed. There was enough space for the abutment teeth 33, 43, 44 inside the lower denture base, which was made using the gypsum dummy of the magnetic assembly (Fig 10).

The magnetic assembly was placed squarely on the keeper (Fig 11). For the abutment 33, a magnetic attachment with 600gf attractive force was set, and magnetic attachments with 400gf were set for the abutment 43, 44. Thus the lower overdenture achieved retentive force of 1,400gf. The applied magnetic assemblies (Magmax) were all coated with adhesive resin, except for the attractive surface. With this coating, there is no need for sandblasting the magnetic assembly nor for applying metal primer on the surface. This issue is a significant feature of the magnetic attachment so as not to have problems with detachment of the magnetic assembly from the denture base.

Next, the fit test material was applied to the denture base and the denture was lightly pressed in the patient's mouth by hand. The fit of the denture and adequate space to place the magnetic assembly on the denture were then checked (Fig 12).

Beforehand, the spill way should be drilled into the lingual side of the polished denture surface where the magnetic assembly is set. The space of the denture base was slightly filled with self-curing resin, and then the lower denture was immediately placed in the patient's mouth with adequate pressure by hand.

After curing the resin, the denture was removed from the patient's mouth and the magnetic assembly checked to insure that it was firmly fixed to the denture base (Fig 13). The complete upper overdenture and the lower overdenture with magnetic attachments was then finished (Fig 14).

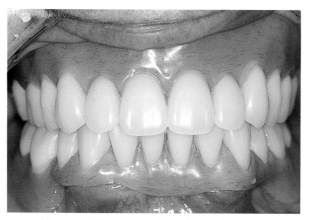

Fig 14 Upper and lower overdenture in oral cavity.

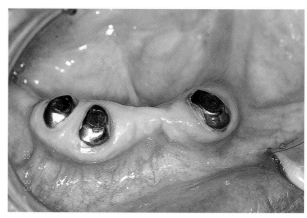

Fig 15 The marginal gingiva of abutment teeth is kept the good condition.

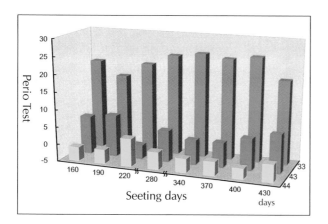

Fig 16 The result of the periodontal index (Perio Test) for all abutment teeth.

Outcome of Treatment

Over the course of one year and three months, the lower overdenture showed adequate retentive force and stability. Thus the mastication function of the patient with the overdenture was well achieved. The marginal gingival of the abutment teeth were also kept in good condition by brushing well (*Fig 15*). Mobility of the abutments was observed in terms of the PI (Periodontal index, *Fig 16*). As seen in the graph, mobility of the abutments did not change greatly for 430 days.

And now anterior hyperfunction syndrome is not observed.

In the case of a few remaining lower anterior teeth, magnetic attachments for overdentures have a beneficial effect on mastication and long-term conservation of the abutment teeth. The reason is that magnetic attachments protect the periodontally weakened abutments from harmful lateral force.

(Hiroshi Inoue)

Case 18
Improvement of Crown-Root Ratio of Abutments—2

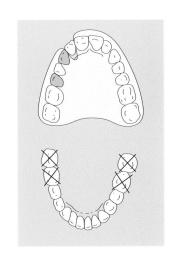

Patient: 69 years old, male

Chief complaint: Fracture of the upper denture

Remaining teeth: 12, 13, 15, 31−35, 41−45

Location of magnetic attachments: 13, 15

Reasons for use of magnetic attachment: Improvement of crown-root ratio

Initial Situation

The patient complained of frequent freature of the upper denture. The denture had broken many times, and there were many cracks in it. The patient wore only the maxillary denture.

He was a constant bruxer and his occlusal force seemed very large. Occlusal surfaces of remaining teeth were considerably worn (*Fig 1*). The teeth of 13 and 15 exposed this roots above gingiva with large crown-root ratios.

The patient wanted to have robust upper denture with a metal base. He missed all lower molars, but refused to wear lower denture.

Treatment Planning and Procedures

In order to improve the crown-root ratio, 13 and 15 were to be used as the root capped abutment with magnetic keeper. These roots were expected to provided periodontal support and retention for the denture by using the magnetic attachment system. Magnetic keepers were aligned face with the axis of the roots. 12 was not used as an abutment tooth for the denture.

13 and 15 were decoronated and prepared for the root cap. Magnetic attachments Hicolex Super J 4015 and 3015 with diameter of 3 and 4mm were selected for 15 (*Fig 2*).

After cementing the root caps, impression for the denture was made. Stone replicas of the magnetic assemblies were mounted on the root caps

of the master cast. The portions of the retentive framework around root caps were opened to leave room for the magnetic assemblies.

Magnetic assemblies coated with adhesive resin Super-Bond C&B were seated on the root caps. The room for the magnetic assemblies of the denture was filled with autopolymerizing resin and the denture was placed in the mouth. After the resin cured, excess was trimmed and polished (*Fig 3*). The denture gave patient aesthetic satisfaction without clasp (*Fig 4, 5*).

Outcome of Treatment

After 4 years, the denture was broken at the retentive framework near the magnetic assemblies. 15 swelled from inflammation and moved. He did not come for recall visit over 4 years span. Because of the residual ridge resorption, root caps were compressed than the mucosa and were in overloaded. The framework surrounding the magnetic assemblies was bended by the occlusal force and the acrylic resin denture base was loosed from the frame.

Then, 15 was extracted and the new denture was to be made. This was designed to reinforce the framework surrounding the magnetic assembly.

Stone replicas of the magnetic assemblies were mounted on the root caps of the master cast (*Fig 6*). The metal framework completely covered over the magnetic assembly and added retention beads were added on the surface (*Fig 7*). The lin-

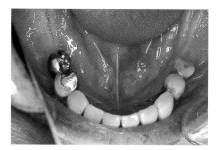

Fig 1 The lower remaining teeth. Occlusal surfaces of the teeth were worn.

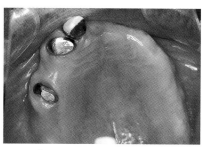

Fig 2 The top of the magnetic keepers are aligned. The circular keeper has a disadvantage for the premolar compared to the oval one.

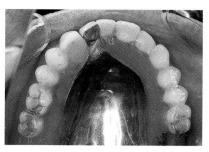

Fig 3 Occlusal view of the upper denture. The lingual surface of 12 was opened. Upper surfaces of the magnetic assemblies were covered only with resin.

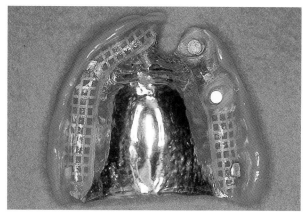

Fig 4 The tissue surface. The magnetic assemblies were covered with autopolymerizing resin, which must not overflow over the surfaces of magnetic assemblies.

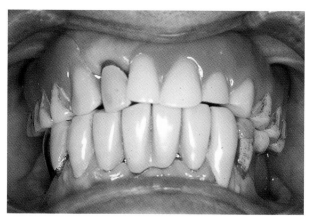

Fig 5 Frontal view.

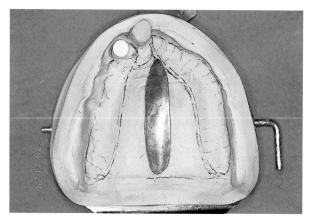

Fig 6 Master cast. Relief of elevated median palatal raphe and stone replica of magnetic assembly were added on it.

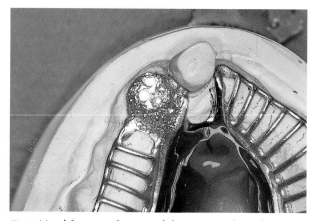

Fig 7 Metal framework covered the stone replica of magnetic assembly and connected with palatal plate.

gual portion of 12 was opened (Fig 8–10).

The patient was instructed to come for recall visit in order to check up the denture and the remaining teeth, and he did every 6 months. The denture was relined every year. He has had a good outcome in the course of 4 years.

When the denture shows tilting movement, the magnetic assembly separates easily from the keeper and the roots are prevented from the overload. But if the denture does not fit the ridge well enough because of the residual ridge resorption, the root were compressed than the ridge.

As the magnetic assembly attaches the keeper at the flat surfaces, the occlusal force is directly

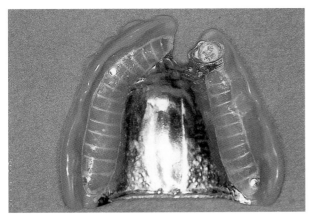

Fig 8 Mucosal view of the denture. The lingual portion of 12 was opened. Magnet assembly was not yet mounted in the housing.

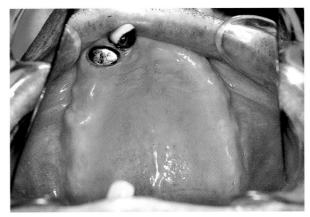

Fig 9 Occlusal view of maxilla. No Inflammation is present around remained teeth.

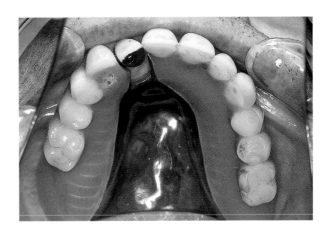

Fig 10 Metal framework over the magnetic assembly was transparent through resin base.

conveyed to the root through the denture and sometimes acts as a torque effect. This compressive torque effect will cause damage to the root.

Thus, the periodic check-up and reline are essential to have a good prognosis.

(Kazuo Nakamura)

Case 19
Improvement of Crown-Root Ratio of Abutments—3 (Cement bonded system)

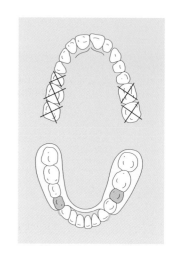

Patient: 69 years old, female

Chief complaint: Dysfunction of mastication

Remaining teeth: 11–14, 21–25, 31–33, 35, 41–44

Location of magnetic attachments: 34, 35

Reasons for use of magnetic attachments: Improvement of crown-root ratio

Initial Situation

The patient visited the clinic with complaints on pain during chewing and bleeding gums. The dental arches were restored by fillings, crowns and bridges though her 36, 37 edentulous area was left as it was (*Fig 1*). Clinical and radiological examination revealed localized advanced periodontitis with severe bone resorption in teeth 34, 36, 37, 40, 47. All these teeth having showed mobility of III degree, were unable to be utilized in support of denture and were subjected to extractions. The upper metal bonding porcelain bridge 11–13, 21–23 was in adequate condition: good fitting, no caries, acceptable esthetics and was left for follow-up.

Treatment Planning and Procedures

A new removable denture restoring lower arch should provide appropriate amount of support, stability and retention. The presence of anterior teeth in lower and adequate length and bone support of 35, 44 teeth permitted application of root caps with bracing option. Combination of conical root cap and magnetic attachment allows achieving good retention and stability of prosthesis as well. Moreover amount of bracing can be controlled through height and taper of root cap and retention by selecting magnetic attachment with particular attractive force. This unique feature is possessed only by magnetic attachments,

as other types of retainers cannot deliver constant retentive force either in initial, or in later periods. After fabrication and fitting of root caps for 35, 44 teeth, the cement bonded Hyperslim 3513 keepers were attached by means of Super-Bond C&B and cemented by the same type of cement (*Fig 2*). According to this cement bonded system, since the keeper is not heated in the furnace at all, the magnetic property of the keeper, such as anti-corrosion, attractive force, etc, is much better than that of cast bonded keeper. However, the matter of concern is longitudinal changes of adhesive force between keeper and metal cap, in another word, removal of keeper from root cap. Lower partial overdenture from acrylic resin reinforced by metal frame was fabricated and inserted in the mouth (*Fig 3a, b*). Magnetic assemblies were embedded by pick-up technique. Patient was instructed regarding hygiene and maintenance of the overdenture.

Outcome of Treatment

After 3.5 years the root caps were fitting well and scratching of keeper surface or corrosion was not detected (*Fig 4a*). Also there were no signs of cement loss around keepers. Upper restorations were still in good condition (*Fig 4b*) and lower denture was stable during function and kept retention unchanged (*Fig 4c*). Radiographs of abutments haven't shown any changes in periapical tissues during service time of denture (*Fig 5a, b*). The patient was satisfied with use of

Fig 1 Frontal view of the mouth upon presentation.
Fig 2 Root caps with cement bonded keepers were set on 35, 44 roots.

1 | 2

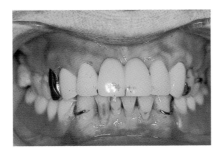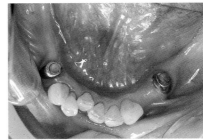

Fig 3a, b A new lower magnetic denture was set in the mouth.

Fig 3a Frontal view of the mouth.
Fig 3b Occlusal view of the lower. The lingual plate was utilized for the major connector.

a | b

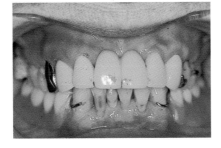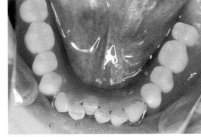

Fig 4a–c Three and a half years after insertion of the the denture setting.

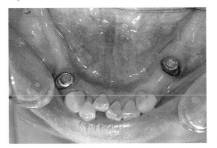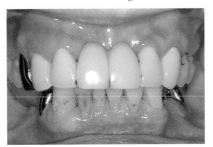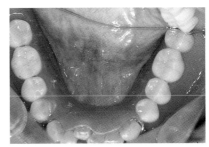

Fig 4a The cement bonded keepers didn't detach from the metal caps at all during this periods. No signs of corrosion and inflammation were observed.

Fig 4b Upper bridge was in good condition.

Fig 4c Occlusal view of the lower denture.

Fig 5a, b X-ray photos 3.5 years after the denture setting.

a | b

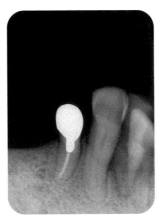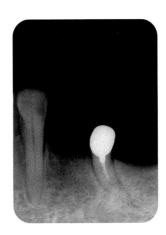

Fig 5a 44.
Fig 5b 35. Bone level of both abutments were still kept and in good condition.

lower partial overdenture and is still under follow-up.

(Hiroshi Mizutani / Vygandas Rutkunas)

Case 20
Reinforcement of Stability of Upper Denture—1

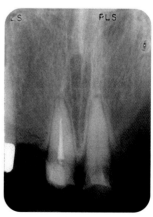

Patient: 72 years old, female

Chief complaint: Instability of former dentures

Remaining teeth: 11, 13, 17, 21, 31–34, 41–43

Location of magnetic attachments: 11, 13, 21

Reasons for use of magnetic attachments: misalignment of anterior teeth, path direction difference between denture insertion and anterior teeth roots and crown-root ratio.

Initial Situation

The patient complained about quality of mastication, speech and esthetics with her former denture. The stability was poor and artificial teeth were considerably worn, therefore it was decided to make new upper and lower dentures. The 17 tooth was restored with cast coping and was overlaid with the former denture base. The marginal fit was satisfactorily good and no caries or periodontal disease revealed (*Fig 1a*).

13 crown showed poor marginal fit, caused plaque accumulation and was removed. Endodontic treatment of upper 13 was successful and no signs of periodontal disease were found (*Fig 1b*). Upper teeth 11, 21 were grossly affected

by caries and demanded endodontic treatment (*Fig 1c–2*). The lower teeth were in proper condition and no pre-treatment preparation except scaling was done (*Fig 3*).

Treatment Plonning and Procedures

As upper 11, 13, 21 teeth were misaligned and were subjected to increased occlusal linguo-labial force from lower natural teeth, it was decided to cut them to gingival level and apply magnetic attachments: More beneficial path of insertion and crown-root ratio was thought to be achieved. Root caps with cast bonded Hicorex slim 4013 keepers were cemented on 11, 21 teeth and with Hicorex slim 3513 keepers on 13. Upper overdenture with full palatal coverage was fabricated (*Fig 4b*). Construction of lower RPD involved lingual bar and incisal continuous bar, wrought wire clasp on 43 tooth and restless Akers

Fig 1a–c X-ray photos on first visit.

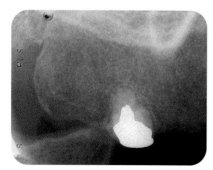

Fig 1a 17 Proper margin fit was observed.

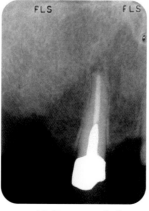

Fig 1b 13 Proper endodontic treatment points but poor margin fit were observed.

Fig 1c 11, 21 Caries were observed and endodontic treatment were needed.

Fig 2 X-ray photos of 11, 21 teeth after endodontic treatment.
Fig 3 Lower occlusal view.

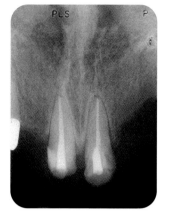

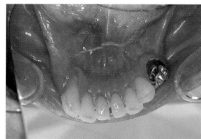

2 | 3

Fig 4a–c New upper and lower dentures.

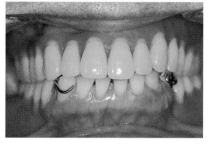

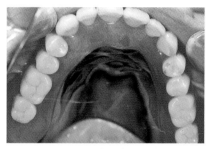

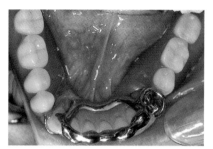

Fig 4a Frontal view of the mouth with the dentures.

Fig 4b Upper occlusal view with the denture.

Fig 4c Lower occlusal view with the denture.

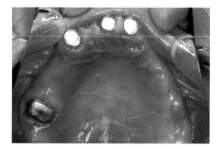

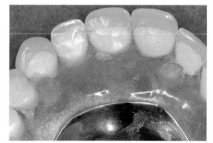

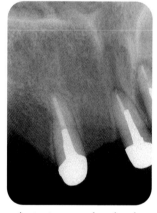

Fig 5 Upper occlusal view without dentures. Magnetic assemblies were embedded in the denture 1 year after the denture setting since the mucosa around 11, 13, 21 was inflamed and needed to be tissue conditioned.

Fig 6 The upper denture one year after insertion of the denture. Location differences between the root caps and the artificial teeth were easily observed.

Fig 7 X-ray photo 4 years after the denture setting.

clasp on 34 tooth (Fig 4c). The dentures were inserted and balanced occlusion created. As appropriate retention of upper overdenture could be achieved even without embedding magnetic assemblies, the overdenture without magnetic attachments aid in tissue conditioning (Fig 5).

Outcome of Treatment

Following 1 year only 2 magnetic assemblies, which provided adequate retention, were applied on 13, 21 teeth (Fig 6). The keeper on 11 teeth was left without retentive function, but aided in support of denture and as a reserved abutment tooth if any of upper abutments would fail. Patient was instructed on proper hygiene of teeth and denture. After 4 years the upper abutments were without signs of periodontal disease, thought minor bone resorption was noticeable (Fig 7).

(Hiroshi Mizutani/Vygandas Rutkunas)

Case 21
Reinforcement of Stability of Upper Denture—2

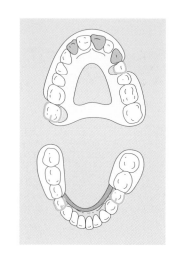

Patient: 69 years old, female

Chief complaint: Pain of 13 tooth

Remaining teeth: 11–13, 17, 21–25, 31–35, 41–44

Location of magnetic attachments: 12, 21, 23

Reasons for use of magnetic attachments: To improvement crown-root ratio and resistance to strong occlusal stress from opposing natural lower anterior teeth.

Initial Situation

The patient visited the clinic with complaint of toothache during mastication and insertion and/or removal of upper denture (*Fig 1*). During intraoral examination, the upper 13 percussion pain and increased mobility were observed. The radiograph showed considerable bone loss and dramatic vertical root fracture (*Fig 2*).

Treatment Planning and Procedures

Nevertheless condition of 11–13, 21, 23 bridge looked good clinically, it was removed due to this fracture. The 11, 13 teeth were extracted. The 23 tooth crown was damaged by caries and endodontic treatment was indicated (*Fig 3*). The tooth 21 had enough alveolar bone and was judged to be utilized for the metal cap abutments though the apex was resorbed. The upper 12, 21, 23 teeth were prepared for metal cast root caps and the polivinylsyloxane impression was taken. The wax patterns of root caps were made and cast-bonded keepers corresponding to size and form of root cap's occlusal area were selected. Thus Hicorex slim 3513 was applied to 12 tooth and Hicorex slim 4013 - to 21, 23 teeth (*Fig 4*). After fitting the root caps, the cast-bonded keepers were cemented on 12, 21, 23 teeth by resin cement.

Super-Bond C&B (*Fig 5*). Though the 25 tooth was considered as a potential abutment initially, it was decided to be extracted since the caries reached 7mm below the level of the gingival margin. Construction of upper denture involved: the ring clasp on 17 tooth, back-action clasp on 24 tooth and posterior strap-type major connector (*Fig 6a, b*). Lower removable partial denture had wrought wire clasps on 35, 44 tooth with cast bracing arm and lingual bar (*Fig 7*). Occlusal pattern with group function was created. Patient was instructed on proper hygiene and denture maintenance.

Outcome of Treatment

One year after treatment, the mobility of abutments have not increased and all restorations had a good marginal fit, though the marginal levels of the abutments went decreased (*Fig 8*). Also vertical space was very limited, where only magnetic attachments can be available especially for 21 tooth. Two years after treatment, the radiograph of abutments didn't show progress of periodontal disease though (*Fig 9*). The upper anterior denture flange was designed to ensure natural cleaning of precervical area of abutments, where gingival inflammation and/or secondary caries is usually located (*Fig 10*). The retention, stability and function of dentures were adequate and patient was satisfied with dentures.

(Hiroshi Mizutani／Vygandas Rutkunas)

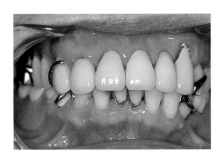

Fig 1 Frontal view of the mouth upon presentation.

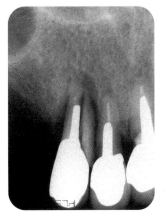

Fig 2 X-ray photo of 13 tooth. Clinically unobserved fracture was clearly taken.

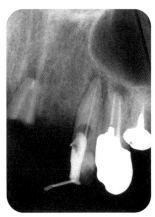

Fig 3 X-ray photo of 21, 23, 24 teeth. The tooth 21 was judged to be utilized for the metal cap abutments though the apex was resorbed.

4 | 5

Fig 4 Wax patterns with keepers on the working cast. The surfaces of the keepers not always have to be parallel, which is one of the advantage of the magnetic attachment.

Fig 5 Three metal caps were set in the mouth. 25 tooth was extracted immediately after these sets.

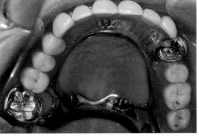

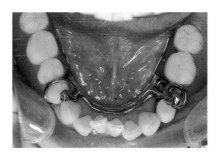

a | b

Fig 6a, b New dentures 3 months after set in the mouth.
Fig 6a Occlusal view of upper denture.
Fig 6b Occlusal view of lower denture.

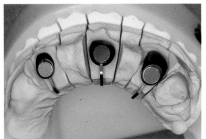

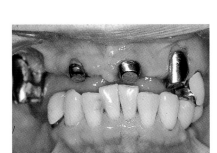

Fig 7 Frontal view of the mouth 1 year after the denture setting. The marginal levels of the abutments went decreased.

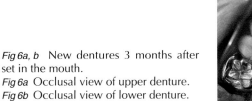

Fig 8 X-ray photo of 12, 21 teeth 2 years after the denture setting. The root apex resorption of 21 tooth was not advanced compared to the 'before treatment stage'.

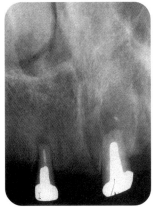

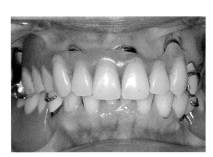

Fig 9 Frontal view of the mouth 2.5 years after the denture setting.

Case 22
Improvement of Poor Appearance of Lower Denture—1

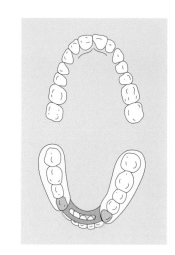

Patient: 66 years old, female

Chief complaint: Instability of lower.

Remaining teeth: 11–17, 21–27, 31–33, 41–44

Location of magnetic attachments: 33, 44

Reasons for use of magnetic attachments: Esthetically good appealing and restricted inter occlusal space.

Initial Situation

The patient addressed the clinic complaining on quality of lower denture. The denture was instable and occlusal surface of artificial teeth was grossly worn, which resulted in instability of denture, discomfort and insufficient mastication. Also the lower 33, 44 abutments were affected by caries. As a consequence of denture base "sinking", the vertical occlusal dimension was decreased and the upper incisors subjected to be overloaded (*Fig1*).

Treatment Planning and Procedures

The patient complained that the clasps on the previously used removable partial denture were visible hence it was decided to fabricate partial overdenture retained by 33, 44 abutments. The 44 tooth have already treated endodontically, thus only the root canal of 33 tooth was treated and obturated by gutapercha (*Fig2*). The 33, 44 abutments were prepared for receiving root caps. During waxing up the root caps, the appropriate sizes of magnetic attachments were selected. In this case two Hicorex Slim 3513 magnetic attachments were applied. The keepers were attached to wax patterns, which were cast with Pd-Ag-Au alloy. The root caps were cemented on abutments by means of Super-Bond C&B adhesive resin (*Fig3*). The lower overdenture design involved the Kennedy's bar type major connector and short hooks approaching labial surface from distal side on 32, 43 teeth for gaining higher stability of denture. This denture was inserted in the mouth and group function occlusal scheme ensured (*Fig4*). At the same time, upper metal bonding porcelain bridge was fabricated and cemented in the mouth (*Fig5*). Since mechanical retention alone was acceptable for the patient, insertion of magnetic assemblies were postponed in order to allow conditioning of soft tissues. Four months after the denture setting in the mouth, the magnetic assemblies were embedded in the acrylic denture base by means of auto-polymerizing resin (*Fig6*). Therefore the retention and support of partial overdenture was considerably increased as well as patient satisfaction. Patient was educated on abutments and denture hygiene and a visit for every 3 month were scheduled.

Outcome of Treatment

In the radiograph taken 3 years after treatment, the absence of carious lesion, proper marginal fit and no bone resorption could be observed (*Fig7*). Four years after the denture setting in the mouth, the 44 artificial tooth was broken and it was replaced by metal cast crown with acrylic facing, which prevents from fracture of artificial tooth in the future (*Fig8*). The denture was also rebased in the laboratory. Thus the denture was very stable and she was satisfied with it.

(Hiroshi Mizutani／Vygandas Rutkunas)

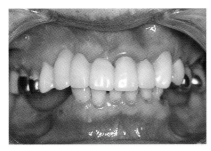

Fig 1 Frontal view of the mouth upon presentation. Upper anterior teeth was a resin-made temporary bridge.

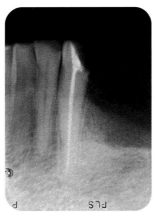

Fig 2 X-ray photo of endodontically treated lower 44 tooth.

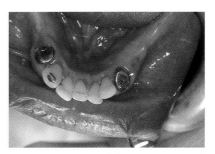

Fig 3 Metal caps with keepers cemented on the lower 33, 44 teeth.

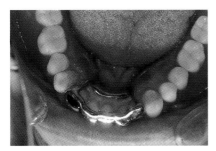

Fig 4 A new fabricated lower denture immediately after set in the mouth.

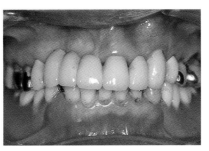

Fig 5 Frontal view of the mouth immediately after the denture setting. Upper Metal Bonding Porcelain bridge was also cemented.

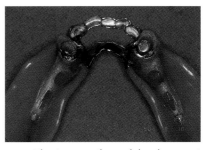

Fig 6 The inner surface of the denture 4 months after treatment. The magnetic assemblies were embedded in the acrylic denture base for the first time.

7 | 8

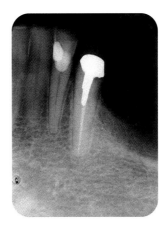

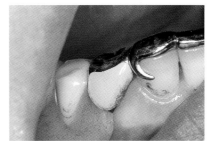

Fig 7 X-ray photo of the 4 tooth abutment 3 years after the denture setting.
Fig 8 Four years after the denture setting in the mouth. The 44 artificial tooth was replaced by metal cast crown with acrylic facing. The denture was also rebased in the laboratory.

Case 23
Improvement of Poor Appearance of Lower Denture—2

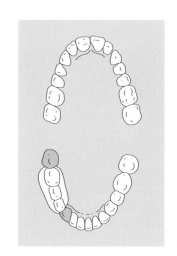

Patient: 45 years old, female

Chief complaint: Poor denture fitting

Remaining teeth: 11–17, 21–24, 27

Location of magnetic attachments: 43,47

Reasons for use of magnetic attachment:

Improvement of the appearance of the lower denture

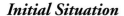

Initial Situation

The patient complained of looseness and poor appearance of the lower denture. The missing teeth were restored with unilateral removable partial denture. The rests were damaged and the denture was displaced toward the mucosa. The residual ridge was narrow and heavily resorbed. 43 and 47 were restored with resin jacket crowns. The upper teeth opposed to the lower denture were supererupted (*Fig1,2*). The patient was unsatisfied with the denture as to its bad fitting and appearance.

Treatment Planning and Procedures

The patient refused to wear a denture with clasps and also disagreed to prepare sound teeth any more. Distance between 43 and 47 was too long for fixed partialdenture supported by only 43 and 47. Then, the to restoration using removable partial denture with magnetic attachments was proposed. 43 and 47 were used as abutment teeth, which were planned to be telescope crowns with magnetic attachments. 43 was to restore as a facing crown.

Artificial crowns of 43 and 47 were removed and both teeth were prepared for inner telescope crowns (*Fig3*). A magnetic keeper was fixed to the top surface of each crown (*Fig4*). Inner crowns were taken in the impression for the outer crowns and the denture (*Fig5*). Outer crowns

and metal framework were made on the master cast. Before the waxing up of the outer crown, the stone replica of the magnetic assembly was added on the magnetic keeper of the inner crown to give space for the magnetic assembly. Axial wall of the inner and outer crowns satisfied the requirement for bracing and some support. Support mainly came from the top surface of the inner crown through the outer crown. Retention was mainly provided from magnetic attachment. The outer crown of 47 with metal framework and the crown of 43 were tried for fitting and secured each other temporally with pattern resin in the mouth. Then they were soldered (*Fig6*). The outer crown of 43 was faced with indirect composite resin. After the denture was cured and polished, the housing of the outer crown (*Fig7,8*) and magnet assemblies were sandblasted. The magnet was bonded in the outer crowns with metal adhesive resin Super-Bond (*Fig9*). New denture filled the requirement for the stability and aesthetics (*Fig10–12*).

Outcome of Treatment

With the passing of 4 years, the denture shows a good resulf now. Magnet retention was stable and the surface of magnetic assemblies and keepers were kept smooth.

Magnetic attachment system always provides fixed attractive force when the magnet assembly and the keeper are in the right place. This is useful to apply the magnetic telescope system for the

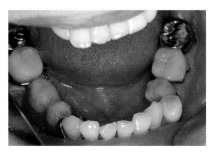

Fig 1 43 and 47 were restored with resin jacket crown. Rests of the denture were broken and the denture settled down to the ridge.

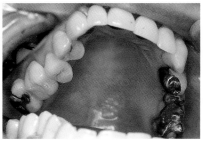

Fig 2 Antagonists of the denture were supererupted.

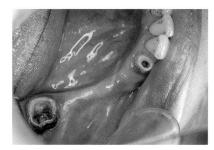

Fig 3 43 and 47 were prepared for the inner crown.

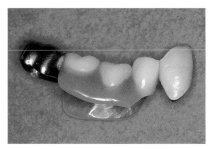

Fig 4 Inner crowns of 43 and 47. Gum contour was duplicated with silicone impression material. Each crown was set a magnetic keeper on its top surface.

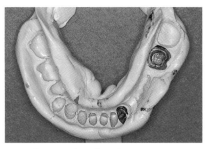

Fig 5 Impression for the outer crowns and the denture. Inner crowns were picked up in the impression.

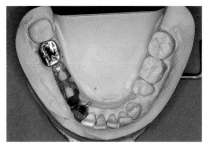

Fig 6 Outer crowns and the metal framework were secured each other temporally with pattern resin.

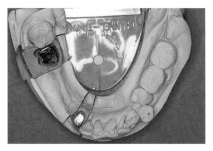

Fig 7 Side view of the denture. The outer crown of 43 was faced with indirect composite. Mandibular new denture. 44, 45, 46 were lost and 47 was restored with metal crown.

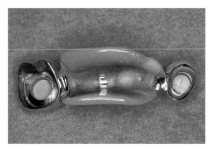

Fig 8 The housing of the outer crown was sandblasted with Al_2O_3 powder.

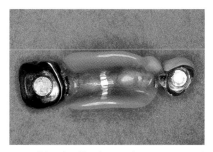

Fig 9 Metal adhesive resin was poured in the housing and seated onto the magnetic assembly coated with metal adhesive resin attached on the magnetic keeper. Then the magnetic assemblies were mounted in the denture.

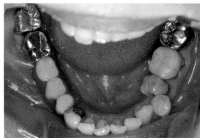

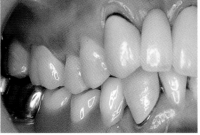

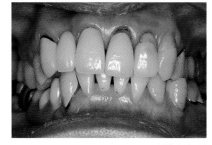

Fig 10–12 New denture satisfied the requirement for the stability and aesthetics.

10 | 11 | 12

removable partial denture. But it is not so easy to bond the magnet assembly in place. Bonding procedure determines the feasibility of the magnetic telescope system.

(Kazuo Nakamura)

Case 24
Improvement of Instability and Poor Appearance of Upper Denture

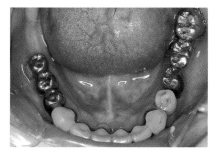

Patient: 81 years old, female

Chief complaint: Instability of denture and esthetically unappealing

Remaining teeth: 11–14, 17, 22, 27, 28, 31–37, 41–46

Location of magnetic attachments: 11–13, 22

Reasons for use of magnetic attachments: Preservation of periodontal tissues, Esthetically good appealing , Easy insertion and removal denture in addition to easy maintenance.

Initial Situation

The patient complaining of instability, bad retention and poor esthetic appearance of upper denture was examined and treated (*Fig 1a~c*). Unfavorable condition resulting from unsuccessful previous treatment was RPD with inadequate support and stability. Upper teeth were subjected to excessive occlusal load of natural teeth and fixed restorations in the lower arch.

Treatment Planning and Procedures

Conditions of 11–14, 17, 27, 28 teeth roots were evaluated radiologically (*Fig 2a~d*) and as the periodontal statuses of 14, 27 teeth were not suitable to provide minimal denture support and had not favorable long-term prognosis they were extracted. The upper partial overdenture was

indicated: the magnetic attachments on 11–13, 22 as an aid for preservation of abutments, relevant retention and esthetics in anterior region; circumferential Akers clasps on 17, 28 to ensure support and bracing in posterior region. Due to palatal tori U-shaped major connector was used.

Carious tissues in 11–13, 22 were removed and roots prepared for root cap restorations (*Fig 3*). The wax patterns of root cap restoration were fabricated in the laboratory and cast-bonded keepers were incorporated into them (*Fig 4*). Particular type and brand of magnetic attachment was selected paying attention to the outline of root cross-section, thus 12, 13, 22 received oval Magfit 400 and 11 circular Hicorex Slim 4013. If outline form of magnetic attachment corresponds with cross-sectional form of the root more powerful magnetic attachment with higher attractive force could be employed. However only to get maximum available retention from each root can not be the main guideline. If it is possible the balanced retention on both sides of

Fig 1 Dental condition upon presentation.

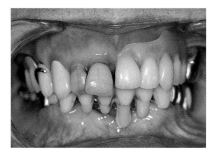

Fig 1a Frontal view.

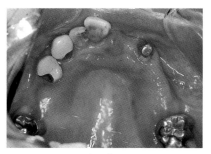

Fig 1b Upper occlusal view

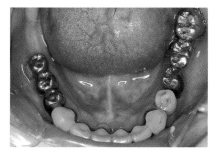

Fig 1c Lower occlusal view

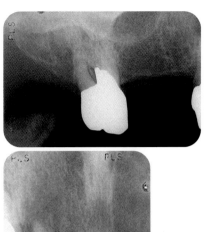

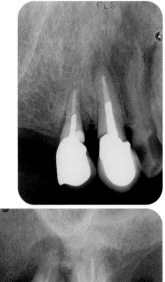

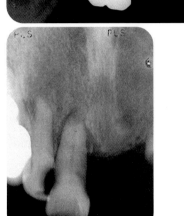

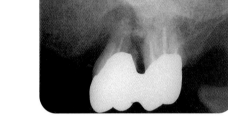

a | b
c | d

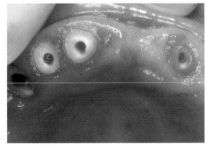

Fig 3 11–13, 22 roots prepared for root caps.

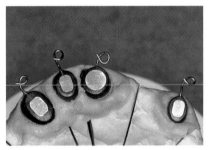

Fig 4 Wax patterns with cast-bonded keepers.

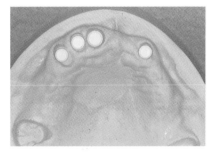

Fig 5 Gypsum dummies on the working model. They are evenly larger than real magnetic assemblies respectively.

6 | 7

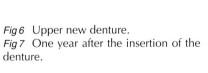

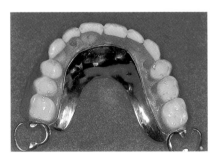

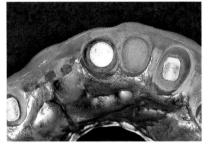

Fig 6 Upper new denture.
Fig 7 One year after the insertion of the denture.

8 | 9

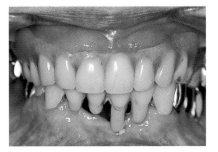

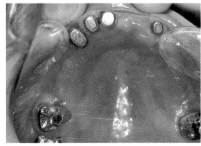

Fig 8 Three years after the insertion of the denture.
Fig 9 Five years after the insertion of the denture.

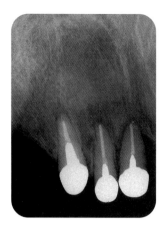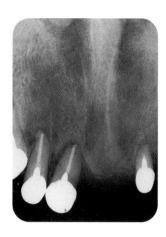

Fig 10a, b X ray photos of lower 11–13, 22 roots five years after the denture setting.

a | b

the arch should be achieved. The keepers were cast-in with Pd-Ag-Au alloy and cemented in usual manner on 11–13, 22 roots. Impressions were taken and old denture was relined for temporarily use. During fabrication of new denture gypsum dummies were used to leave even space for auto polymerizing acrylic resin around magnetic assemblies (*Fig5*). This is useful because unevenly distributed auto polymerizing resin around magnetic assembly is often caused to removal of magnetic attachment. Therefore attractive force (retention) will be reduced. Newly made RPD was inserted and the magnetic assemblies were embedded into acrylic base with auto polymerizing acrylic resin (*Fig6*). Patient was instructed on proper hygiene of dentures and abutments and follow-up visits.

Outcome of Treatment

One year (*Fig7*), three years (*Fig8*) and five years (*Fig9*) after treatment, the upper denture was still in good condition and magnetic attachments were not corroded and post treatment care was limited mainly to relining and minor occlusal adjustment. There were no complications with root caps on 11–13, 22 teeth and the retentive force remained constant. Radiographs of 11–13, 22 teeth didn't show any signs of peri-apical lesions (*Fig10*).

(Hiroshi Mizutani／Vygandas Rutkunas)

Case 25
Application of the Root Keeper System

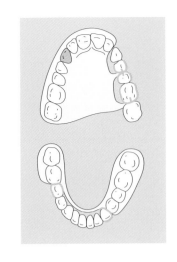

Patient: 67 years old, female

Chief complaint: Uncomfortable chewing and increased mobility of teeth, fracture of upper abutment tooth and loss of denture retention

Remaining teeth: 13–15, 23–27, 31–33, 41–45

Location of magnetic attachments: 13

Reasons for use of magnetic attachments: Immediate (Fast) denture repair, favorable crown-root ratio

Initial Situation

The patient referred to clinic with complains about upper denture. Examination revealed advanced periodontitis with bone resorption in 14, 15 teeth and resultant vertical mobility of them. Coronal part of 13 tooth was fractured, thus upper RPD lost its retention and stability. It was decided to repair the present denture and fabricate a new partial overdenture. However she had to go abroad and wanted us to repair the denture immediately.

Treatment Planning and Procedures

14, 15 teeth were not able to utilize as abutments and were extracted. The day after extraction of 14, 15 teeth, root of 13 tooth was prepared for the magnetic attachment abutment (*Fig 1*) to protect 13 tooth from detrimental lateral forces and gain favorable crown-root ratio. The Root keeper which has 800 gf retentive force, estimated by manufacturer was selected (*Fig 2*). The root canal

was prepared (*Fig 3*) and the keeper was try-in position (*Fig 4*) in order to check the keeper surface angle in relation to the occlusal plane, comparative position to the root tooth, and so on. Then the keeper was cemented by DC Core (Kuraray, Japan) dual (light and chemical) cure resin cement (*Fig 5, 6*). The pre-existing denture was rebased and the magnetic assembly was embedded in it (*Fig 7*). The patient was very pleased with this repaired denture. Two years after repairing the denture, a new upper partial overdenture and a lower RPD were fabricated and inserted (*Fig 8*). The patient was satisfied with retention and stability of the new dentures. The lower teeth required splinting and meticulous hygiene.

Outcome of Treatment

Regarding the 13 root tooth covered with dual cure resin, the follow-up showed the satisfactory results after 3 years. The changes in periodontal condition of 13 abutment after 3 years have not been occurred (*Fig 9a, b*). Also any signs of corrosion of magnetic assembly or keeper were not seen and retention properties remained unchanged after

1 | 2

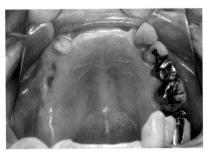

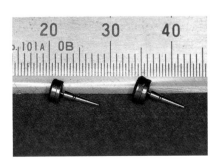

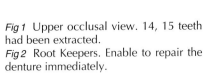

Fig 1 Upper occlusal view. 14, 15 teeth had been extracted.
Fig 2 Root Keepers. Enable to repair the denture immediately.

169

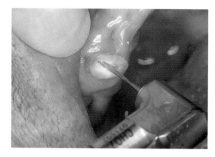

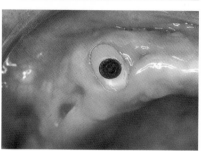

Fig 3 Preparation of root canal.
Fig 4 A root keeper was try-in into the 13.

3 | 4

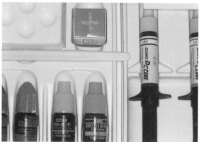

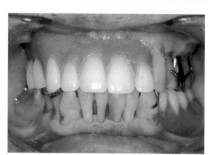

Fig 5 Dual (light and chemical) cured resin cement DC Core.
Fig 6 The keeper was cemented and the resin cap was polished.

5 | 6

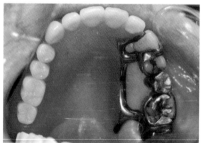

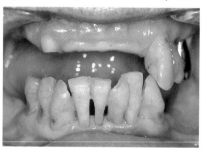

Fig 7a, b Rebased and magnet attached pre-existing denture.

a | b

Fig 7a Mucosal surface with magnetic assembly.
Fig 7b Mucosal surface with magnetic assembly.

Fig 9a, b Three years after resin cap with root keeper (13) was fabricated.

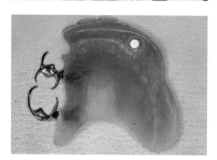

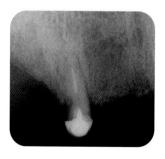

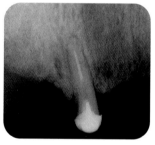

Fig 8 A new upper partial overdenture set in the mouth.

Fig 9a Frontal view of the mouth without the denture.

Fig 9b X-ray photo.

Fig 10a, b Four years after resin cap with root keeper (13) fabrication.

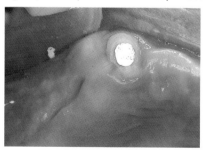

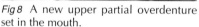

a | b

Fig 10a 13 abutment tooth. Disto-palatal side of the resin cap was broken.
Fig 10b X-ray photo. Secondary caries was suspected because of fracture of resin cap.

4 years, though minor scratching of keeper surface could be noticed (Fig 10a). Radiograph of 3 tooth performed after 4 years have not revealed periapical bone resorption, however precervical caries due to insufficient hygiene on distal side was suspected (Fig 10b).

(Hiroshi Mizutani／Vygandas Rutkunas)

Case 26
Application for Implant Supported Lower Denture—1

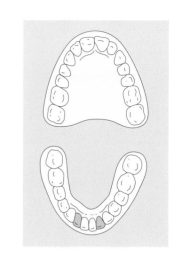

Patient: 74 year old, female

Chief complaint: Masticatory disturbance due to instability of mandibular denture

Remaining teeth: Fully edentulous

Location of magnetic attachments: 32, 42

Reasons for use of magnetic attachments: Advanced bone resorption, implant-supported overdentures, minimal intervention

Initial Situation

The patient was wearing complete dentures fabricated about 5 years ago for both upper and lower jaws. The denture stability was very poor due to advanced resorption of the alveolar bone. In the mandible, in particular, she was suffering from pain and numbness due to the interference of the denture with mental nerves. The patient strongly desired denture stabilization by means of implant therapy.

Treatment Planning and Procedures

Although there was nothing particular in her medical history, we decided to use only 2 implants to minimize surgical invasiveness, taking into account her age. Advanced bone resorption in her mandible not only forced us to use shorter implants, but also indicated difficulties in attaining ideal insertion positions and/or directions of the implants.

For such a patient, magnetic attachments were excellent solution, because of the capability to break the harmful lateral force exerted on the denture, and there is less restriction when detaching the denture in any direction.

We classified magnetic attachment applications into the following 3 categories, according to the functional roles: Type R (the functional pri-

ority is placed on retention, not on suppor or bracing); Type SR (the main purpose is support and retention, not bracing); and Type BSR (bracing, support and retention are equally expected).

In the case of this patient, as aforementioned, the bone volume was very poor and only 2 implants were used. As a result, we selected Type R prosthetic design, by placing the priority on breaking the harmful lateral force, in order to protect the 2 implant abutments that were to be inserted into a severely atrophied alveolar bone.

In addition, we decided to place implants in anterior regions where a lesser load on occlusal support is expected.

Implant surgery with minimal incisions and ablations was carried out. In contrast with other attachments, magnetic attachment can compensate for some inaccuracy in positions and/or angulations of implants. Thanks to this advantage of magnetic attachments, the implant surgery of this patient was comparatively easy, despite the very narrow bone width.

After the healing period, overdentures were fabricated using MACS System, which is a magnetic attachment system with a pre-mounted resin cap on the denture magnet. After the denture was fabricated using the standard procedure, a small amount of self-curing resin was applied to the hollowed-out sections of the mucosal aspect of the denture, and the denture was fit to the magnet with the resin cap in the patient's mouth. Because the purpose of this step was the position-

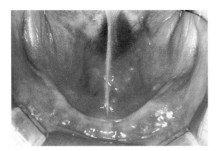

Fig 1 Initial situation. Advanced bone resorption is apparent.

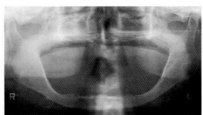

Fig 2 Panoramic radiograph at the time of first visit indicates that the mental foramen is positioned at the alveolar crest due to the advanced bone resorption.

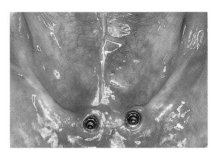

Fig 3 Placed only 2 implants (ITI Bonefit® 4.1, 10mm long) in the lateral incisor regions to minimize surgical invasiveness.

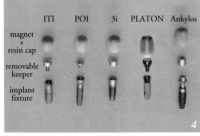

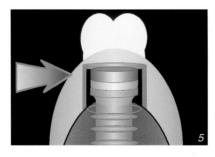

Fig 4 The magnetic attachment used for this patient was MACS System. This system has a resin cap pre-mounted on the magnet.
Fig 5 The clearance provided between the keeper and cap of the MACS System allows easy fabrication of denture designed to break harmful lateral force on abutments.

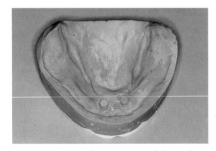

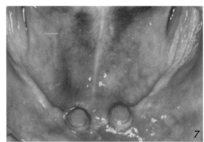

Fig 6 Intraoral view. Removable keepers are mounted on the implants after successful osseointegration.
Fig 7 After the fine adjustment of the margin of resin caps, the denture magnet with pre-mounted resin cap was connected to the removable keeper, and an impression was taken.

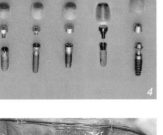

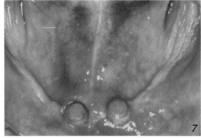

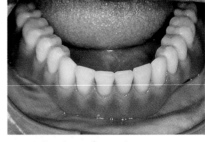

Fig 8 Completed master model. A denture was fabricated using the standard procedure, the magnet position on the mucosal aspect of the denture was hollowed-out slightly deeper in order to make space to accommodate the self-curing resin for magnet connection.

Fig 9 A small amount of self-curing resin is applied to the hollowed-out section on the mucosal aspect of the denture, and the denture is fit to the magnet *in situ*.

Fig 10 Because the resin cap prevents the self-curing resin from flowing into undercuts, the denture can be left long enough for the resin to cure completely without any risk of difficulties in removing the dentures after polymerization.

ing of the resin cap and the hollowed-out section only, a very small amount of self-curing resin was enough and there was no need to create a channel to release excessive resin.

In addition, the pre-mounted resin cap prevented self-curing resin from flowing into under-

cuts. After the resin cured, the denture was removed and the small gap between the margin of the resin cap and the hollowed-out section on the mucosal aspect of the denture was retouched with a thin brush. Thus, the magnet denture could be fabricated in a simple and easy manner.

Fig 11 After the resin cures, the denture is removed to retouch the small gap between the resin cap margin and the hollowed-out section of the denture using a thin brush.

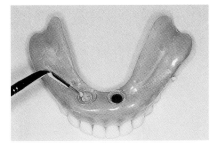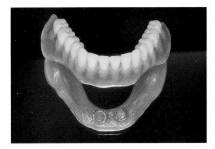

11 | 12

Fig 12 Completed magnet denture. The clearance provided between the resin cap and keeper can prevent harmful lateral force exerted on denture from being directly transmitted to implant abutments.

Fig 13 Although a relief was made at the area of mental nerves, magnetic attachments facilitate high denture stability. Treatment outcome, including the masticatory function, esthetic, comfort and ease of handling and cleaning, is satisfactory.

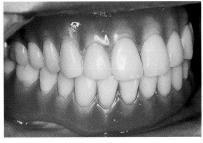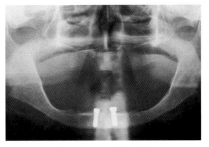

13 | 14

Fig 14 Post-surgical panoramic radio-graph. Although the patient was very old, use of magnetic attachments capable of compensating for inaccurate positions and/or angulations of implants facilitated comparatively easy implant surgery with minimal invasiveness. Treatment outcome is quite satisfactory.

Outcome of Treatment

A relief was made on the denture to avoid the interference of the denture and the mental nerves. The magnetic attachments allowed excellent stability of the denture, leading to the recovery of masticatory function. The treatment outcome, including high denture stability, esthetic, comfort, and ease of use and cleaning, was satisfactory. The clearance provided between the resin cap and keeper, which is one of the unique advantages of MACS System, facilitated easy fabrication of Type R restoration, by avoiding direct transmission of the harmful lateral force onto the implant abutments.

Bar attachment is one of the typical retainers used for implant-supported overdentures. Bar attachments require splinting of implants, which results in disadvantages such as difficulties in fabricating passive-fit prosthesis and the need of implantation at optimal locations and accurate angulations. In particular, the cases with severely atrophied V-shaped alveolar ridge are contraindications of bar attachments, due to the risk of interference with tongue space.

When compared with other stud attachments, magnetic attachments have greater advantages such as no risk of attenuation of retaining force during long-term use, excellent capability of breaking the harmful lateral force and less restriction on the detaching direction.

(Jyoji Tanaka)

Case 27
Application for Implant Supported Lower Denture—2

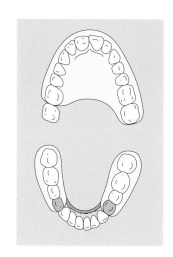

Patient: 55 years old, female

Chief complaint: Mobility of teeth provided with clasps

Remaining teeth: 11–17, 21–27, 31–33, 41–44

Location of magnetic attachments: 34, 44

Reasons for use of magnetic attachments: Mobility, esthetic restoration, remaining root, minimal intervention

Initial Situation

In the mandible of the patient, teeth from 45–47 and 34–37 were missing, and there was a remaining root in location 44. The patient was wearing partial dentures for 44–47 and 34–37. Simple wire clasps were provided to the left and right lower canines, and these teeth showed mobility while chewing food. The main complaints of the patient were worrying about the excessive load on these clasped teeth and esthetic problems resulting from these clasps.

The mobility of the left and right lower canines was about M_2, and redness and swelling were apparent in the proximal to lingual regions of the gingiva around these teeth. The periodontal pocket depth around these 2 canines was greater than 5mm, and as deep as 8mm at the proximal regions. The remaining root in 44 showed mobility of about M_1, and the periodontal pocket depth around the root was approximately 4mm.

Treatment Planning and Procedures

The treatment option included the primary stability, by means of splinting of the remaining anterior teeth, and the secondary stability, by means of conus crowns. However, all the remaining teeth 33–43 were vital and the aforementioned treatment option was not considered optimal in light to the minimal intervention concept.

Although the patient accepted implant treatment, we selected magnetic attachment prosthesis using only 1 implant, which is placed in 34, as the abutment. This solution can effectively cope with the restrictions in terms of both the anatomical condition of the alveolar ridge and the economical condition of the patient. We also decided to use the remaining root in 44 as the abutment of magnetic attachment, based on the judgment that the magnetic attachment structured to break the harmful lateral force can effectively protect the root with M_1 mobility. We selected MACS System that uses removable keeper, to avoid interference with an MRI examination in the future.

In order to meet the strong needs of the patient for esthetic improvement, as well as to minimize the load on the left and right canines, a non-clasp denture was planned. Denture coloring was used for the denture base to attain a highly esthetic outcome. Clear resin was used for the margin of the denture with an expectation of a "chameleon effect" so that the boundary between the denture base and the natural gingiva is unclear.

Outcome of Treatment

Magnetic attachment solution using an implant and remaining root successfully improved the denture stability and resolved the masticatory disturbance. Esthetic improvement by means of non-clasp structure attained great

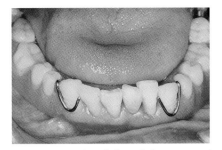
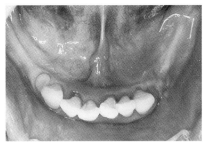

Fig 1 Initial situation. The patient is wearing old dentures. The main complaints were worrying about the excessive load on the left and right canines and esthetic problems due to clasps.

1 | 2

Fig 2 Pre-surgical intraoral view. Remaining root in 44, and mobility of about M_2 at the left and right lower canines.

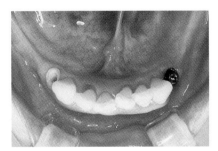
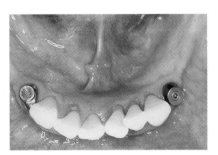
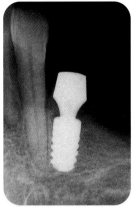

Fig 3 In light to minimal intervention concept, no treatment was provided to the remaining anterior teeth of the mandible. The remaining root in 44 and the implant placed in 34 are used as the abutments.

Fig 4 Intraoral view after the connection of removable keepers. Surgical invasiveness was minimal because magnetic attachments allow the use of a shorter implant.

Fig 5 Radiographic evaluation of implant at 34. Removable keeper is connected to the implant abutment (Ankylos Implant ø4.5, 8mm long).

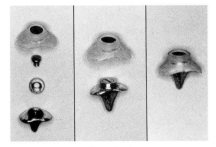
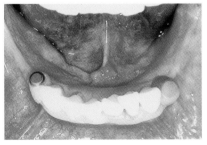
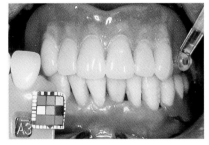

Fig 6 For natural teeth abutment, MACS System (Inoue Attachment, Japan) provided with measures for MRI is used.

Fig 7 Magnet with resin cap is mounted. Impression is taken and the denture is fabricated using the standard procedure.

Fig 8 For highly esthetic outcome, photos for shade definition are taken using denture shade and Cas Match (Kyowa Tokei Kogyo, Japan) and sent to the laboratory.

satisfaction from the patient.

The mobility of the left and lower canines reduced, the redness and swelling of the gingival mucosa disappeared, and the pocket depth decreased to about 3mm in all regions around the canine teeth. The mobility of remaining root in 44 was also reduced and the pocket depth became less than 3mm. The implant replacing the first premolar indicated excellent prognosis.

Implants were originally used for fixed bridges. Today, however, implant-supported overdentures have become popular, thanks to the advantages such as good lip support, phonetics, ease of cleaning, cost effectiveness, esthetic and

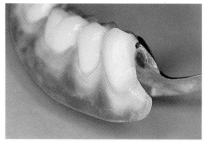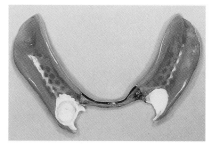

9 | 10

Fig 10 Completed denture. In order to secure the space for self-curing resin for magnet connection, the gap between the hollowed-out section and the resin cap was confirmed using a fit-checker (GC, Japan) in the patient's mouth.

Fig 9 Clear resin was used for the margin of the denture with an expectation of the "chameleon effect" so that the boundary between the denture base and gingival mucosa is unclear.

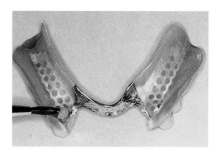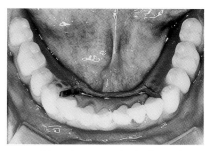

11 | 12

Fig 12 The denture fits to the magnet in the patient's mouth. It should be noted that the magnet might slide off if the denture is removed before the resin completely cures.

Fig 11 In order to accurately position the magnet with resin cap to the hollowed-out sections of the denture, only a small amount of self-curing resin should be applied to the hollowed-out sections and the denture is fit to the magnet in the patient's mouth.

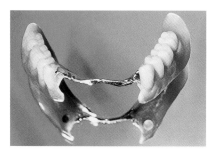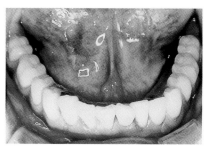

13 | 14

Fig 14 Intraoral view with completed magnet denture. Denture stability is excellent and the mobility of the left and right canines is improved. Highly esthetic and comfort to use prosthetic restoration achieved the improvement of QOL of the patient.

Fig 13 The small gap between the resin cap margin and the hollowed-out section of the denture is retouched with a small amount of self-curing resin. Thus, the magnet overdenture is fabricated in a simple and easy procedure. Denture coloring is used also for the denture base for esthetic improvement.

comfort of use. Nonetheless, most of the implant-supported overdentures are for completely edentulous cases and its application to partially edentulous patients is very few, due to the difficulties in terms of both prosthetic design and handling of retainers.

Thanks to the unique advantages, such as retention without bracing, no need of splinting, ease of conjunctive use with natural teeth, less restriction of position and/or angulation of implantation, and the small-size and ease of maintenance, the application of magnetic attachments to partially edentulous patients is simple and easy. Use of magnetic attachment will facilitate implant therapy for a wider range of indications.

(Jyoji Tanaka)

Materials: Dental magnet attachments which are sold in Europe and USA

Products	Type	Maker	Country	Magnetic structure	Magnetic assembly		
					Diameter (mm)	High (mm)	Magnetic structure
Magfit	DX 400	Aichi Steel Corp.	Japan	Closed cap	3.4	1.0	Material Magnet: Nd-Fe-B Yoke: 19Cr-2Mo-Fe stainless steel
	DX 600				4.0	1.2	
	DX 800				4.4	1.3	
	RX				4.4	1.4	
Dyna WR Magnet	S3	Dyna Dental Engineering	Nether lands	Opened cap	4.7	1.7	Magnet: Nd-Fe-B Case: Non-magnetic material
	S5				4.7	2.7	
Titanmagnetics	X-Line	Steco system tecknik	Germany	Opened cap	4.8	2.65	Magnet: Sm-Co, Case: Ti
	Z-Line				5.8	3.15	
	K-Line				5.2	5.0	
	T-Line				5.8	5.7	
Micro Plant	—	Gebr. Brasseler GmbH	Germany	Opened cap	4.4	3.15	Magnet: Nd-Fe-B Case: Ti
Magna-Cap	Mini	Technovent	U.K.	Closed sandwich	4.5	3.2	Magnet: Nd-Fe-B Yoke: Magnetic material Case: Ti
	Midi				5.5	3.2	
	Maxi				5.5	3.9	
Micromagnet	Mini	Redeim	France	Closed cap	4.4	1.7	Magnet: Nd-Fe-B Yoke: 30Cr-Fe stainless steel
	Small				4.8		
	Medium				5.2		
	Large				5.6		
Shiner Smart Magnet System	—	Preat Corp.	USA	Closed sandwich	5.5	3.4	Magnet: Nd-Fe-B Yoke: Magnetic material

Attractive force (N)	Remarks	Coping method	Keeper			Height in Total (mm)	Attractive force performance (N/mm3)
			Diameter (mm)	High (mm)	Material		
3.9	Laser welding, Dome shaped attractive face, Wing	Cast	3.0	0.5	19Cr-2Mo-Fe stainless steel	1.5	0.31
6.3		Cast, Root Keeper	3.6	0.7		1.9	0.28
7.7		Cast, Root Keeper	4.0	0.8		2.1	0.26
		Implant	4.7	1.4		2.7	0.17
6.0		Root Keeper	4.4	1.0		2.2	0.18
		Implant	4.7	1.6		2.8	0.13
2.9	Laser welding	Cast	—	—	Pd-Co Alloy	—	—
		Root Keeper	4.7	1.5		3.2-4.2	0.05-0.07
		Implant	4.7	3.0		4.7-5.7	0.04-0.05
4.9				4.0		5.7-6.7	0.03-0.04
				5.0		6.7-7.7	0.02-0.04
1.7	Laser welding, Dome shaped attractive face, Self centering	Root Keeper	4.8	2.5	Magnet: Sm-Co, Case: Ti	5.15	0.02
		Implant	4.8	4.0		6.65	0.01
3.0			5.8	4.4		7.55	0.02
1.6			5.2	5.6		10.6	0.01
1.4			5.8	8.2		13.9	0.01
1.5	Sand-blasted	Implant	3.8	3.2	Magnetic material	6.35	0.02
				4.2		7.35	0.02
				5.2		8.35	0.01
4.0	Dome shape magnet, Wing	Cast Keeper	4.4	0.8	Magnetic material	4.0	0.09
			5.1	1.1		4.3, 5.0	0.07
6.2		Root Keeper	4.4	1.1		4.3	0.09
			5.4	1.1		4.3, 5.0	0.08
7.2		Implant	5.4	3.8		7.0, 7.7	0.05
2.0	Laser welding, Anti-rotation milled	Cast Keeper	4.4	0.6	30Cr-Fe stainless steel	2.3	0.06
2.9			4.8				0.07
3.9			4.8				0.08
4.9			5.6				0.09
6.6	Resin cap, Stepped keeper	Root Keeper	4.0	1.4	Magnetic material	4.8	0.07
		Implant	4.0	1.0		4.4	0.07

INDEX

A

adhesive resin cement ···················· 50, 65

advantage and disadvantage of the

magnetic attachment ·················· 67

altered cast technique ···················· 63

alternating magnetic field ················ 44

animal biocompatibility test ············· 42

anode polarization test ··················· 40

air gap ································· 36, 37

arrangement of the magnetic attachment ········· 68

artificial saliva test ······················· 41

AUM20 ···················· 27, 36, 38, 39, 40, 41, 42, 86

autopolymerizing resin ············· 120, 126, 140, 145, 162

B

biocompatibility ························· 42, 83

biological effect of magnet assembly ·········· 45

bone remodeling ······················· 47

bracing ········· 58, 59, 63, 65, 66, 67, 71, 72, 73, 74, 98, 99,

111, 116, 120, 156, 160, 164, 176

B-H curve ···························· 31

C

cap-type ··························· 28, 36, 54

cardiac pacemaker ···················· 19, 48

cast-bonded keeper system ··············· 72, 73

cementaion of keeper ··················· 72

cement-bonded keeper technique ········ 75, 79, 82, 83, 84

closed circuit ·············· 18, 20, 33, 75, 79, 82, 83, 84

corrosion ··········· 16, 19, 20, 23, 24, 28, 29, 31, 36, 37, 38,

39, 40, 41, 51, 53, 55, 56, 75, 76, 82, 85,

86, 123, 138, 140, 148, 156, 169

crown-root ratio ············ 70, 98, 125, 132, 133, 134, 149,

153, 156, 158, 160, 169

CR ratio ······························ 123

cup-yoke type ························· 19

Coulomb's Law ························· 32

cumulative survival curve ················ 93, 94

Curie point ··························· 38

Curie temperature ······················ 24

custom made keeper ···················· 74

D

Dalla Bona spherical attachment ············· 111

dental alloy ························· 75, 76

denture base ········· 16, 17, 24, 26, 27, 59, 60, 61, 63, 64, 66,

68, 71, 72, 76, 84, 88, 95, 111, 122, 125,

137, 140, 141, 151, 153, 158, 162

divesting and pickling ··················· 80

dome-shaped attractive face ··············· 51

dual-cure composite resin cement ············ 86

E

endodontic consideration ················· 71

extrusion ···························· 149

F

ferromagnetic alloy ···················· 75

finishing and polishing ················· 78, 82, 83

flat attractive face ····················· 51

4-META resin ························· 86

G

galvanic corrosion test ··················· 42

Gillings ························· 17, 34, 85

H

holder ························· 28, 30, 52

housing pattern ······················ 79, 83

hygiene ············· 57, 70, 87, 97, 111, 120, 140, 143, 146,

156, 159, 160, 162, 167, 169

hygiene of overdentures ·················· 103

I

immersion test ························ 40

implant ··············· 19, 22, 30, 44, 51, 71, 97, 171, 174

implant abutment connection ·············· 25

implant prosthodontics ·················· 22

incorporated cast keeper ················· 51

indication for the RK system ·············· 87

indirect retainer 68, 120

inter-dental brush 71, 104

inter occlusal space 121

investment and casting 81

K

Kaplan-Meier method 93

keeper 19, 24, 28, 45, 48, 51, 61, 72, 75, 85, 93,
100, 109, 111, 114, 116, 118, 120, 123,
125, 127, 129, 132, 134, 137, 140, 143,
146, 150, 153, 156, 158, 164, 166, 169,
173, 174

keeper selection 79

keeper setting 79

M

MACS system 171, 174

Magfit 28, 50, 51, 86, 93, 109, 114, 116, 118,
123, 127, 137, 140, 146, 166

Magfit-IP 53

magnet 16, 22, 28, 44, 48, 51, 58, 70, 75, 85, 93, 97,
109, 111, 114, 116, 118, 120, 123, 125, 127,
129, 132, 134, 137, 140, 143, 146, 149, 153,
156, 158, 160, 162, 164, 166, 169, 171, 174

magnet location 26

magnetic assembly 19, 28, 45, 51, 61, 82, 86, 100,
114, 120, 123, 125, 132, 134,
139, 140, 143, 150, 153, 164,
167, 169

magnetic attachment 16, 22, 25, 44, 48, 51, 58, 70,
75, 85, 93, 97,109, 111, 114,
116, 118, 120, 123, 125, 127,
129, 132, 134, 137, 140, 143,
146, 149, 153, 156, 158, 160,
162, 164, 166, 169, 171, 174

magnetic attractive force 30

magnetic circuit 28, 45, 55

magnetic field 18, 23, 31, 32, 33, 38, 44, 45, 47,
48, 85, 103

magnetic flux 18, 29

magnetic flux leakage 18, 34

magnetic force 30, 31, 32, 38, 86, 92

magnetic risonance imaging (MRI) 48

magnetic retention 23, 38, 56, 91

magnetization characteristic 31

maintenance of overdentures 97

major connector 59, 111, 160, 162, 166

Maxwell's equations 33

micro-laser welding 29, 39, 53, 99

minor connector 59

MRI 19, 27, 44, 48, 52, 85, 104, 174

N

Neodymium-Iron Boron (NdFeB) 28

neodymium-iron magnet 19

nickel allergie 42

north pole 30

O

occlusion 27, 58, 100, 118, 125, 145, 159

open circuit 17, 33, 51

overdenture 20, 23, 30, 44, 61, 70, 71, 76, 80, 84, 87,
90, 92, 97, 98, 99, 100, 101, 102, 103,
104, 105, 109, 110, 111, 114, 120, 122,
126, 129, 134, 140, 143, 145, 146, 147,
148, 149, 150, 151, 152, 156, 157, 158,
159, 162, 169, 171, 173, 175, 176

overdenture design 97, 98, 162

P

pacemaker 19, 48, 50, 103

patient satisfaction 97, 98, 99, 142, 162

possible risks of the RK system 88

prefabricated keeper 75

preservation of residual ridges and abutments 97

pressure impression technique 61

protection of abutment teeth 60

proximal plate 59, 62

R

rare-earth magnetic material ·················· 85, 86

relining, rebaseing and remaking of the overdentures

··· 101

removable partial denture ············· 20, 23, 57, 81, 118,
120, 127, 129, 135,
160, 162, 164

repair of denture ······························· 67

rest ······································ 22, 62, 90, 132, 137, 164

retentive force ·············· 18, 19, 20, 23, 28, 29, 51, 59, 61,
64, 66, 68, 75, 99, 100, 109, 140,
151, 152, 156, 169

retention ·············· 16, 19, 22, 23, 24, 25, 28, 40, 56, 58, 59,
62, 63, 65, 66, 68, 70, 71, 76, 78, 79, 86,
87, 88, 91, 92, 93, 98, 99, 102, 105, 109,
111, 113, 114, 117, 118, 119, 120, 121,
123, 125, 127, 129, 132, 134, 137, 140,
141, 146, 153, 156, 159, 160, 162, 164,
166, 168, 169, 176

rigid-support ································· 60

root cap ····················· 19, 40, 52, 71, 75, 85, 99, 109, 111,
116, 118, 120, 125, 128, 129, 132,
134, 137, 140, 143, 146, 150, 153,
156, 158, 162

root cap design ··························· 71, 76

root coping ······························ 73, 76, 99

root keeper ·························· 25, 51, 63, 85

root keeper installation ···················· 25

root keeper system ······················ 63, 85

root surface attachment ·················· 16, 61, 109

S

samarium-cobalt magnet ···················· 18

sandwich type ····························· 86

sandwich-yoke type ······················ 18, 19

self-curing resin ···················· 20, 95, 102, 150, 173

short root length ························ 129, 132

silicone gum imitation ······················ 76

single tooth brush ························· 103

spruing ································· 80

south pole ······························· 30

special care for the RK system ················ 90

spin ································· 130

Sm-Co$_5$ magnets ························· 129

static magnetic field ······················· 44

stud attachment ························· 109, 173

super thin magnetic attachment ················ 56

support ··················· 16, 22, 30, 50, 53, 57, 70, 90, 97, 118,
120, 129, 134, 137, 146, 153, 156,
159, 162, 164, 166, 171, 176

SUS304 ································ 39

SUS316 ······························ 28, 86

T

telescope crown ·········· 56, 59, 78, 114, 116, 119, 134, 164

telescope system ························ 18, 164

troubleshooting ························· 103

tray-in keeper system ····················· 72

V

vertical space ·················· 23, 71, 84, 104, 109, 120

W

wax pattern ··············· 75, 114, 134, 150, 160, 162, 166

with Root Keeper system ···················· 72

Y

yoke ································ 18, 28, 86